ABC OF SPORTS AND EXERCISE MEDICINE
Third Edition

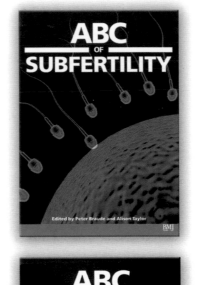
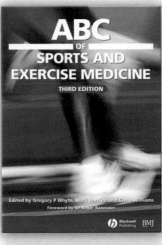
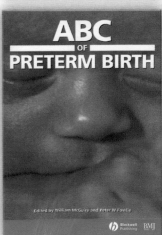

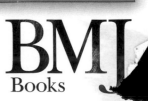

ABC OF SPORTS AND EXERCISE MEDICINE

Third Edition

Edited by

GREGORY P WHYTE
*Olympic Medical Institute, Northwick Park Hospital,
Harrow, Middlesex*

MARK HARRIES
*Olympic Medical Institute, Northwick Park Hospital,
Harrow, Middlesex*

and

CLYDE WILLIAMS
*Professor of Sport and Exercise Science,
University of Loughborough*

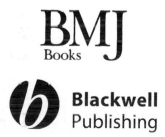

BMJ
Books

Blackwell
Publishing

© 1995, 2000 BMJ Books
© 2005 by Blackwell Publishing Ltd
BMJ Books is an imprint of the BMJ Publishing Group Limited, used under licence

Blackwell Publishing, Inc., 350 Main Street, Malden, Massachusetts 02148-5020, USA
Blackwell Publishing Ltd, 9600 Garsington Road, Oxford OX4 2DQ, UK
Blackwell Publishing Asia Pty Ltd, 550 Swanston Street, Carlton, Victoria 3053, Australia

First published 1995
Second edition 2000
Third edition 2005

Library of Congress Cataloging-in-Publication Data
ABC of sports and exercise medicine/edited by Gregory P. Whyte, Mark Harries, Clyde Williams.— 3rd ed.
      p. ; cm.
   Rev. ed. of: ABC of sports medicine/edited by Greg McLatchie ... [et al.]. 2nd ed. BMJ Books, 2000.
   Includes bibliographical references and index.
   ISBN-13: 978-0-7279-1813-0
   ISBN-10: 0-7279-1813-3
  1. Sports medicine.
   [DNLM: 1. Sports Medicine. 2. Athletic Injuries. 3. Exercise. QT 261 A134 2005]
 I. Whyte, Gregory P. II. Harries, Mark. III. Williams, Clyde. IV. ABC of sports medicine.

   RC1210.A24 2005
   617.1′027—dc22

                        2005006580

ISBN-10: 0 7279 1813 3
ISBN-13: 978 0 7279 1813 0

A catalogue record for this title is available from the British Library

Set in 9/11 pt New Baskerville by Newgen Imaging Systems (P) Ltd, Chennai, India
Printed and bound in India by Replika Press Pvt. Ltd

Commissioning Editor: Eleanor Lines
Development Editors: Sally Carter, Nick Morgan
Production Controller: Debbie Wyer

For further information on Blackwell Publishing, visit our website:
http://www.blackwellpublishing.com

Contents

Contributors

John Aldridge
Consultant orthopaedic surgeon, Coventry and Warwick University Hospital

Caryl Becker
Rehabilitation manager, Olympic Medical Institute, Northwick Park Hospital, Middlesex

Karen Birch
Senior lecturer in exercise physiology, department of sport and exercise sciences, University of Leeds

Lynn Booth
Consultant physiotherapist to the British Olympic Association

John Buckley
Exercise physiologist and lecturer, school of health and rehabilitation, Keele University and University Hospital of North Staffordshire

Richard Budgett
Director of medical services, Olympic Medical Institute, Northwick Park Hospital, Middlesex

John Dickinson
Research physiologist, Olympic Medical Institute, Northwick Park Hospital, Middlesex

Susie Dinan
Senior clinical exercise practitioner and research fellow, department of primary care and population sciences, Royal Free at University College School of Medicine, London

K Donaldson
Professor of respiratory toxicology, MRC Centre for Inflammation Research, University of Edinburgh Medical School

Geraint Florida-James
Senior lecturer in sport and exercise science, school of life sciences, Napier University, Edinburgh

Colin W Fuller
Lecturer and safety management consultant, University of Leicester

Mark Gillett
Consultant in accident and emergency, department of accident and emergency, Russell Hall Hospital, Dudley

O J A Gilmore
Director and consultant surgeon, The Groin and Hernia Clinic, 108 Harley Street, London

Richard Godfrey
Research lecturer, sports sciences, school of sport and education, Brunel University, Middlesex

Mark Harries
Consultant physician, Olympic Medical Institute, Northwick Park Hospital, Middlesex

Caroline J MacEwen
Consultant ophthalmologist, Ninewells Hospital and Medical School, Dundee

Paul McCrory
Associate professor, Centre for Sport Medicine Research and Education and Brain Research Institute, University of Melbourne, Australia

William J McKenna
Professor of cardiology, cardiology department, Heart Hospital, Wimpole Street, London

Jayesh Makan
Research fellow in cardiology, department of cardiology, University Hospital Lewisham, London

Roger Palfreeman
Director of medicine, British Cycling Federation, National Cycling Centre, Manchester

Geoffrey Pasvol
Professor of infection and tropical medicine, Imperial College, London and Northwick Park Hospital, Middlesex

K R Postlethwaite
Consultant maxillofacial surgeon, Newcastle General Hospital

Sanjay Sharma
Consultant cardiologist, department of cardiology, University Hospital Lewisham, London

Patrick Sharp
Consultant endocrinologist, department of diabetes and endocrinology, Northwick Park Hospital, Middlesex

Nigel Stephens
Consultant cardiologist, Northwick Park Hospital, Middlesex

Vicki Stone
Reader in toxicology, school of life sciences, Napier University, Edinburgh

Mike Tipton
Professor of human and applied physiology, department of sport and exercise science, University of Portsmouth

A D J Webborn
Medical director, The Sussex Centre for Sport and Exercise Medicine, University of Brighton, Carlisle Road, Eastbourne, East Sussex

Gregory P Whyte
Director of science and research, Olympic Medical Institute, Northwick Park Hospital, Middlesex

Clyde Williams
Professor of sport and exercise science, University of Loughborough

Peter Wilmshurst
Chair of the United Kingdom Sport Diving Medical Committee, and consultant cardiologist, The Royal Shrewsbury Hospital

Archie Young
Professor of geriatric medicine, University of Edinburgh

Foreword

Since the success of earlier editions there has been an inexorable rise in the popularity and participation in sport. Equally inexorably, the numbers of injuries have risen. Most sports involve some risk exposure, which young people need and welcome. It is our duty to frame the rules to minimise the risks of injury. If, however, injury occurs, the medical services must be organised to ensure well researched basic sciences of physiology and biomechanics linked to prompt, precise, and effective treatment. The National Health Service will be the usual and most efficient route of delivery.

Sports injuries are best treated in specialised sports injury clinics by doctors with specialist recognition. Until this target is achieved, accident and emergency departments will do the best they can, aided by this book as a guide and friend.

Sport for all should go hand in hand with sports medicine. Sports injuries must be better treated in future. Moreover, the lessons learnt from a skilled and dedicated service will become part of better treatment of other injuries sustained in the community.

There is no clearer, more compact, comprehensive, authoritative manual of sports and exercise medicine. I congratulate the editors, contributors, illustrators, and publishers on a fine achievement. No doctor, physiotherapist, or coach should be without it.

Sir Roger Bannister

1 Epidemiological studies of sports injuries

Colin W Fuller

Most sports have a certain risk of injury; some sports considerably more than others. Although developing effective measures to treat sports injuries and reduce the time that athletes remain injured is important, preventing injuries in the first place is equally important. The risk of injury normally should be controlled by the sports governing body through risk management. This process requires identifying potential risk factors, assessing the level of risk, and implementing control measures that will reduce the risk to an acceptable level. Risk management, however, will be successful only if the decisions made about implementing control measures are evidence based. A high proportion of this evidence comes from epidemiological studies that identify the aetiology, incidence, and severity of injuries to participants in individual sports. To obtain valid data from this source, however, epidemiological study designs must be robust. Issues related to the design of epidemiological studies of sports injuries are discussed below, with examples from football and rugby union.

Study population

Epidemiological studies must define the overall **target population at risk**: the people who would be counted as cases if they had the type of sports injury being investigated. As target populations sometimes are very large, common practice is to define a smaller **sample population** from which the target population is drawn. The confidence that can be ascribed to any conclusions derived from the data obtained from a sample population depends on the sample size and its relation with the target population. Potential errors because of the size of the sample can be quantified and accounted for through statistical analysis. Errors that arise from a poor sampling strategy, however, are more difficult to correct. For example, in a study of osteoarthritis in retired professional footballers (target population) using a postal questionnaire, the respondents (sample population) may be unrepresentative of the target population as ex-players with osteoarthritis may be more likely to respond than ex-players without osteoarthritis.

Statistical power

Epidemiological studies determine whether associations exist between risk factors and incidence of injury. Inferential statistics are used to determine the validity of these associations and to avoid type I and type II errors.

The power of a statistical test is the probability of making the correct decision about an association between a risk factor and the incidence of injury. Failure to achieve an adequate level of statistical power can lead to errors. The power of an epidemiological study can be increased by enlarging the sample population, considering associations with big effects, looking for large differences in the mean values of two sample populations, and accepting a lower level of statistical significance (although the minimum acceptable value is normally 0.05). Ideally, an epidemiological study should have a power of 80%.

Definition of injury

One definition of an injury that would be applicable to all sports would be convenient and simple; however, to reach a consensus view on such a definition is very difficult, if not

Comparison of level of injury in range of popular sports[*]

	Self-reported injuries per 1000 occasions of participation	
Sport or activity	All injuries	Lost-time and substantive injuries
Rugby	96	58
Football	64	20
Hockey	63	14
Cricket	49	14
Badminton	29	7
Squash	24	6
Tennis	23	5
Horse riding	17	5
Running	15	5
Swimming or diving	6	2

[*]Adapted from Nicholl JP, Coleman P, Williams BT. The epidemiology of sports and exercise related injury in the United Kingdom. *Br J Sports Med* 1995;29:232-8

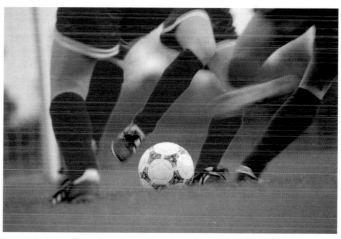

Football and rugby union are team games where injuries often occur and this chapter uses examples of epidemiological studies of both sports

Potential errors in epidemiological studies

Type I error

Results indicate no association between a risk factor and the incidence of injury, when in fact an association does exist

Type II error

Results indicate an association between a risk factor and the incidence of injury, when in fact no association exists

Number of participants needed in sample population in epidemiological studies to detect effects at confidence level of 0.05

	Participants needed to produce percentage size of effect =		
Power of study (%)	20	40	60
20	35	10	10
40	75	20	10
60	125	30	15
80	195	45	20

impossible. Some authors recommend that injuries should be excluded from epidemiological studies if they only need the use of ice and bandaging for treatment. Others argue that even injuries that do not result in lost time could affect an athlete's long term physical and mental condition, and so all injuries that need medical attention should be included in epidemiological studies. An advantage of categorising all player complaints that need medical attention as an injury is that it allows a definition that is applicable to all sports. A disadvantage of this approach is that the inclusion of minor contusions—for example, in studies of some contact sports—could create an overwhelming burden on the healthcare professionals involved. Understanding which injuries are included and which are excluded from a study is essential when reporting or interpreting data.

Injury definitions using lost time are often sport specific—for example, a broken finger would probably cause a rugby union player to miss training and competition but the same injury would be unlikely to limit a footballer's activities unless the player was a goalkeeper. Injuries that result in insurance claims only relate to players that have insurance cover, and injuries definitions using hospital attendance will probably produce data biased towards more severe injuries.

Study design

Effective epidemiological studies can be achieved through a number of study designs. A cohort study measures the effect of a risk factor on the level of injury in a sample population, whereas a case–control study compares the level of injury observed in a sample population exposed to a risk factor with the level in an unexposed population. Cross sectional studies measure the level of injury seen in a sample population at a given time, whereas a longitudinal study measures the level of injury in the same sample population repeatedly over an extended period of time. Retrospective studies collect historical information about a sample population, and prospective studies use data over a future period of time. Prospective epidemiological studies normally produce more reliable data than retrospective studies because respondents have been shown to have poor recall of injuries over even a short time.

Classification of injuries

A suitably qualified medical practitioner should always diagnose sports injuries in the context of epidemiological studies to ensure the validity of the data. The international statistical classification of diseases, injuries and causes of death (ICD), which is published by the World Health Organization, is an internationally recognised classification system used for clinical diagnosis. The system, which uses a three element alphanumeric code to identify the nature of injuries, is not designed specifically for the study of sports injuries. A simpler system for sports injuries is the orchard sports injury classification system, which was developed by Dr John Orchard in Australia (www.sportsinjurymanager.co.uk/osics.html). It also use a three element alphanumeric code, with the first element (a letter) identifying the area of the body injured, the second element (a letter) the pathology, and the third element (a number or letter) the diagnosis of the injury.

Measuring the level of injury

When the number of injuries seen in an epidemiological study is reported the aetiology of the injuries by location and diagnosis can be defined. This allows simple intersport comparisons of injuries to be made.

Definitions of injuries used in epidemiological studies

- Any new injury sustained during training or competition that prevents a player from participating in normal training or competition for more than 48 hours.
- Any injury sustained during a game or practice session that resulted in an insurance claim.
- Any injury that required a player to attend hospital.
- Any player complaint that required post-match medical attention from the team physician.
- Any injury (new or recurrent) sustained during competition that prevented a player from participating in the next match.
- Any injury that restricted the participant from taking part in usual activities, including days off from work.

Orchard sports injury classification system

Body area

Head
- Head (H)
- Neck (N)

Upper limb
- Shoulder (S)
- Upper arm (U)
- Elbow (E)
- Forearm (R)
- Wrist (W)
- Hand (P)

Trunk
- Chest (C)
- Abdomen (O)
- Thoracic spine (D)
- Lumbar spine (L)

Lower limb
- Buttock (B)
- Groin or hip (G)
- Thigh (T)
- Knee (K)
- Lower leg (Q)
- Ankle or heel (A)
- Foot (F)

General
- Multiple areas (X)
- Medical problem (M)
- Area not specified (Z)

Diagnosis
- Common diagnoses identified with digits 1-7
- Diagnoses not in list of common diagnoses use number 8
- Unknown diagnosis uses number 9
- Special diagnoses use letters A-Z

Pathology

Bone
- Fracture (F)
- Avulsion or chip (G)
- Stress fracture (S)
- Old fracture (Q)

Joint
- Dislocation (D)
- Recurrent instability or subluxation (U)
- Chondral, articular cartilage, or meniscal damage (C)
- Minor joint problem with or without synovitis (J)
- Atraumatic arthritis, effusion, joint pain, chronic synovitis, gout, or other rheumatological condition (P)
- Degenerative arthritis (A)
- Ligament tear or strain (L)

Soft tissue
- Muscle tear or strain (M)
- Muscle spasm, cramps, soreness, trigger points, overuse, or myalgia (Y)
- Tendonitis, bursitis, enthesopathy, apophysitis, or periostitis (T)
- Complete rupture of tendon (R)
- Haematoma, bruising, or cork (H)
- Laceration or skin condition (K)

Other
- Developmental abnormality (B)
- Infection (I)
- Tumours (E)
- Visceral damage, trauma, or surgery (O)
- Neural condition or nerve damage (N)
- Vascular condition (V)
- Reflex sympathetic dystrophy (W)
- Systemic disease process (X)
- Undiagnosed (Z)

Comparison of location of injuries in rugby union and football

Injury location	Injuries (%)	
	Rugby union	Football
Head or neck	11	4
Upper limb	17	3
Trunk	12	7
Lower limb	60	86
Total	100	100

If only the number of injuries seen in epidemiological studies are reported, however, limited information about the risk of injury to the sample population can be obtained, as conclusions about risk can be made only if the number of people and length of time they are exposed to a risk factor are taken into account. The two most common measures for reporting the level of injury in epidemiological studies are **incidence** and **prevalence**. Incidence is the number of injuries (new or recurrent, or both) seen in the sample population divided by the total time participants are exposed to a risk factor. Incidences in sports injury studies often are normalised to an exposure period of 1000 hours to allow intersport comparisons. Incidence is the measure that should be used in conjunction with studies of the aetiology of injuries.

Prevalence refers to the proportion of a sample population that is injured at a given point of time (point prevalence) or within a specified time period (period prevalence). Period prevalence is the more appropriate measure for reporting relatively rare chronic injuries, whereas incidence normally should be reserved for reporting acute injuries. Prevalence is related to the product of the incidence and the average severity of injuries. A new injury becomes a case within a measure of incidence and within the current prevalence measurement. The injury only counts once when measuring incidence, however, it remains a case in prevalence measurements until the player has recovered from the injury. Prevalence is often reported as the percentage of a population that is injured.

Measuring the severity of injuries

There have been a variety of definitions used for measuring injury severity in epidemiological studies. It is important, however, to appreciate the full implications associated with each definition. For example, descriptive phrases, such as "minor," "moderate" and "major" can be misleading because some minor injuries that are related to time lost from training and competition can still involve serious tissue damage and may lead to chronic consequences. In addition, different definitions of severity may be more appropriate for amateur and professional sportspeople because, for an amateur sportsperson, the days lost from training or competition, or both, may be zero but the time absent from their normal occupation may be up to a week.

High injury severity values, which imply a slow recovery rate, do not affect the incidence of injury but they do lead to high prevalence values. Similarly, low severity values, which imply a rapid recovery from injury, do not affect the incidence value but in this case they lead to low prevalence values. It is, therefore, essential to report the severity of injuries in epidemiological studies because otherwise a large number of minor injuries may mask the true impact of a small number of major injuries. Multiplying the number and severity of each type of injury enables the risk associated with injuries to be calculated and risk factors to be ranked with regards to their overall importance.

Risk factors and injury incidence

The outcomes from epidemiological studies should include the incidence and severity of injuries as a function of each risk factor, such as training and match play. In this way, the relative importance of each risk factor can be identified and appropriate preventive and therapeutic measures implemented.

Calculation for incidence of injury

A football club plays 96 matches in a season lasting 46 weeks; during this time, the players suffer 42 injuries.

$$\text{Exposure time} = 96 \text{ (matches)} \times 1.5 \text{ (length of match in hours)}$$
$$\times 11 \text{ (number of players in study team on pitch)}$$
$$= 1584 \text{ player hours}$$

$$\text{Incidence} = (42/1584) \times 1000$$
$$= 27 \text{ injuries}/1000 \text{ hours of competition}$$

Calculation for prevalence of injury

A rugby union club has 30 players in the senior squad. During one week, six players are injured and, therefore, are unavailable to play or train.

$$\text{Prevalence} = (6/30) \times 100$$
$$= 20\%$$

Comparison of injury incidence and risk in professional football

Injury diagnosis	Number (%)	Average severity (days)	Total days lost	Percentage risk
Sprains	70 (19.2)	18.7	1310	25.7
Strains	148 (40.7)	12.5	1845	36.2
Contusions	72 (19.8)	7.2	515	10.1
Fractures or dislocations	14 (3.8)	34.2	479	9.4
Others	60 (16.5)	15.8	947	18.6
Total	364 (100)	14.0	5096	100

Comparison of injury incidence and severity as function of injury location and activity in international rugby union

Injury location	Injuries per 1000 hours (severity, days)	
	Match	Training
Head or neck	31 (13)	0.3 (4)
Upper limb	43 (16)	0.6 (8)
Trunk	25 (6)	0.9 (28)
Lower limb	119 (16)	4.3 (13)
Total	218 (14)	6.1 (14)

Further reading

- Drawer S, Fuller CW. Evaluating the level of injury in English professional football using a risk based assessment. *Br J Sports Med* 2002;36:446-51
- Finch CF. An overview of some definitional issues for sports injury surveillance. *Sports Med* 1997;24:157-63
- Fuller CW. Implications of health and safety legislation for the professional sportsperson. *Br J Sports Med* 1995;29:446-51
- Meeuwisse WH. Predictability of sports injuries. What is the epidemiological evidence? *Sports Med* 1991;12:8-15
- Nicholl JP, Coleman P, Williams BT. The epidemiology of sports and exercise related injury in the United Kingdom. *Br J Sports Med* 1995;29:232-8
- Orchard J. Orchard sports injury classification system (OSICS). *Sport Health* 1993;11:39-41
- Van Mechelen W, Hlobil H, Kemper H. Incidence, severity and prevention of sports injuries: a review of concepts. *Sports Med* 1992;14:82-99

2 Immediate care

Mark Gillett

Most pitchside medical staff fortunately will never have to treat a life threatening injury on the field of play. The fact that these situations occur so rarely means that unless specific equipment is available and appropriate training undertaken, they will be ill prepared to deal with such dangerous situations.

Planning phase

Training
Pitchside medics come from many different fields and possess a wide variety of baseline skills and knowledge. The pitchside scenario itself may vary, with large events having dedicated paramedic crews in attendance, together with well trained crowd doctors, whereas smaller community events may have no form of medical cover. Similarly, the expectations of care delivered by the differing professional groups will be markedly different. Doctors reasonably will be expected to treat life threatening injuries and stabilise the casualty before transfer to hospital, while physiotherapists will be expected to possess the skills needed to ensure a clear airway and cervical spine protection under similar circumstances. Often, however, physiotherapists will not have the luxury of a doctor in attendance and may be confronted with a potentially treatable life threatening injury. On this basis, practitioners increasingly are upgrading their skills to ensure patient safety.

The practitioner's duty is to ensure that they are trained to the minimum level expected of their discipline and that their skills are reviewed and refreshed regularly.

Equipment
Despite being appropriately trained, a pitchside medic will be unable to work to the best of their ability if essential items of emergency equipment are not available.

Generally practitioners should carry a selection of airway tubes, a pocket mask, and an adjustable cervical collar as part of their own kit. Supplementary oxygen, spinal boards and an automated external defibrillator should be provided at the venue but to locate these items well in advance of the start time is the practitioner's responsibility.

Response phase

Safety
This should be prioritised in the order: self, scene, and casualty. Although a dramatic injury may inspire acts of heroism, the reality may result in personal injury and thus put the injured player at further risk. This principle is common sense during a high speed sport such as horse racing or cycling, but it also holds true for sports such as football and rugby, where often the game will continue around the injured player. Only when the medic is satisfied that they and others surrounding the scene are at low risk of injury can they attend to the fallen player.

Primary survey
The primary survey follows the ABCDE approach.

Airway management and control of the cervical spine
Airway management remains the major clinical priority in any critical situation, purely because severe hypoxia results in irreversible cerebral damage within three minutes. The principles of look, listen, and feel should be followed.

Phases of immediate care
- Planning
- Response
- Recovery

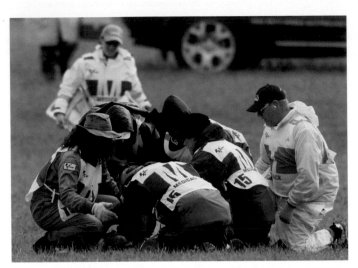

Large events may have a dedicated paramedic crew and smaller events may have no medical cover

---

Equipment list
- Oropharyngeal airways (variety of sizes)
- Nasopharyngeal airways (variety of sizes)
- Pocket mask
- Cervical collar (adjustable)
- Supplementary oxygen supply with non-rebreathable masks
- Spinal board
- Automated external defibrillator

When a player requires immediate treatment there is no time to hunt for equipment

---

Sections of response phase
- Safety
- Primary survey
- Removal from pitch or track
- Secondary survey

Primary survey

A—airway with cervical spine control
B—breathing
C—circulation with haemorrhage control
D—disability
E—environment and exposure

If the injured player seems not to be breathing on initial assessment, the immediate priorities are to open the airway and perform manual in line stabilisation of the head and cervical spine. Jaw thrust is preferred to head tilt as an airway manoeuvre, as it involves less movement of the cervical spine and so reduces the risk of damaging the cervical area of the spinal cord. Ideally, a second rescuer should perform manual in line stabilisation to free up the primary medic to complete the primary survey. If this is not possible, however, the head can be maintained effectively in line by kneeling astride the head and managing the airway from this position. If jaw thrust restores airway patency, consideration can then be given to inserting a nasopharyngeal airway tube or an oropharyngeal airway tube to free the rescuer's hands. Nasopharyngeal airway tubes do not stimulate the gag reflex to the same degree that oropharyngeal airway tubes do, and hence they can be used with a semiconscious person. In all patients who tolerate an artificial airway, high flow oxygen should be administered as soon as possible at the highest possible flow rate.

Breathing assessment

In practice, the patient's airway and breathing are assessed simultaneously. The rescuing medic should observe the casualty for chest wounds and asymmetry of chest movement. The rate and pattern of respiration also are important. Tachypnoea may result from pain but is also an early sign of hypovolaemia, while a significant head injury can lead to an irregular breathing pattern. A tension pneumothorax is seen most commonly secondary to penetrating trauma, but it can on occasion result from closed trauma. If the patient shows clinical features of a tension pneumothorax, then a needle decompression should be performed without delay.

Circulatory assessment

The two crucial assessment tools used for a circulatory assessment are the capillary refill time and the pulse rate. The pulse rate of an injured athlete is often an unreliable indicator of evolving hypovolaemic shock, principally because the pulse rate is likely to be high during sporting activity. The site in which a pulse is able to be palpated can give vital information about the casualty's blood pressure according to the following rule of thumb:

- Carotid pulse palpable: systolic blood pressure > 60 mm Hg
- Femoral pulse palpable: systolic blood pressure > 70 mm Hg.

The capillary refill time is obtained by pressing on the sternum for strictly five seconds before releasing. The skin should return to its normal pink colour within two seconds—any longer than this is suggestive of hypovolaemia. The capillary refill time often is assessed by pressing on the nailbed of one of the exposed fingers; however, vasoconstriction induced by cold weather may give a falsely prolonged refill time.

Disability

Disability refers to the patient's neurological status and relies on an AVPU assessment and pupillary response to light. Pupillary response is an unreliable indicator of raised intracranial pressure in a fully conscious patient. Hence any inequality in the reactivity of the right and left pupils to light in a fully conscious patient is more likely to be due to direct ocular trauma or be a coincidental finding. The classical signs of sluggishly reactive or fixed dilated pupils are late features of raised intracranial pressure and are not compatible with a fully conscious patient

Exposure and environment

Injury can compromise thermoregulatory compensatory mechanisms and put the player at a higher risk of hypothermia

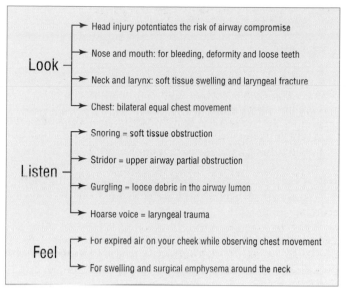

Look, listen, and feel in the primary survey

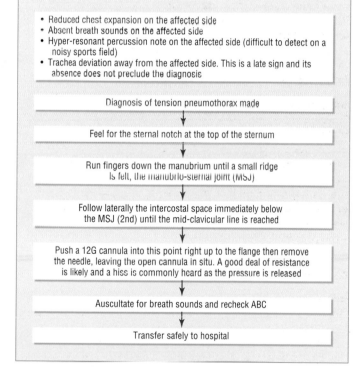

Diagnosis and treatment of a tension pneumothorax

AVPU score

The patient's response level is:
A—alert: able to obey commands and talk coherently
V—verbal: responds to verbal stimuli
P—pain: responds to painful stimuli
U—unresponsive

or hyperthermia, depending on the ambient temperature. Once the patient has been stabilised, the priority becomes removal to an area that is temperature controlled and private to allow full exposure of the injured area.

Removal from the pitch or track

Athletes who cannot have an injury to the cervical spine excluded on the pitch should be placed in a semi-rigid cervical collar and on a long spinal board, with the head immobilised in head blocks. Full protection of the cervical spine encompasses all three of these components, although sandbags or litre bags of intravenous fluid can be used to improvise when head blocks are unavailable. The long spinal board is essentially a transfer device, and the patient needs to be removed from the long board as soon as they have been log rolled and assessed on arrival in the emergency department in order to prevent development of pressure sores.

Vacuum extraction mattresses can be used as an alternative to the long spinal board, and these may be favoured by paramedics in certain areas.

The easiest means of transferring an injured player onto a spinal board involves the use of a scoop stretcher, which can be split into two vertical halves by release bolts at either end. Half of the stretcher then can be placed on either side of the patient, before the bolts are reconnected and the patient lifted onto the spinal board in a controlled fashion. Alternatively, the player can be log rolled onto the board, although four people are needed to perform this properly and it often involves repositioning up and down the board.

Secondary survey

If a player sustains an isolated limb injury, often a formal secondary survey is not needed. In cases of more extensive trauma or when a player sustains a considerable cervical spine or head injury, however, a systematic head to toe clinical evaluation must be performed. This should occur after the player has been stabilised and removed from the pitch, which in practice often does not take place until they arrive in the emergency department.

Recovery

Treatment of a player for a life threatening or limb threatening injury is unusual and stressful for any sports physician. The psychological sequelae should not be underestimated, and they may be profound—regardless of the outcome. Only when the medic feels ready should the incident be discussed and appraised with professional colleagues to decide if performance and procedure could be improved in the future.

Specific categories of injury

Fractures and dislocations

Practitioners should be wary of the potential medicolegal consequences of performing on field manipulations. If a fracture is suspected, the neurovascular status of tissue distal to the injured area should be assessed and recorded. If the distal area is judged to be neurovascularly intact, then the region should be immobilised and the patient transported to hospital for further treatment. Simple splint devices such as the structural aluminium malleable (SAM) splint or box splint are very useful, although for lower limb injuries, simply splinting to the contralateral limb is very effective. If the distal area is judged to be vascularly compromised, with a delayed capillary refill time and absent pulse, gentle realignment may be attempted

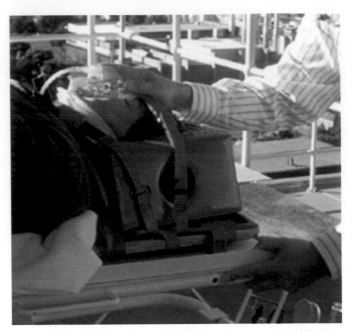

Patient on spinal board—shows semirigid collar, bolsters, and positioning of the straps

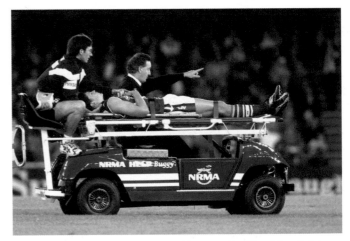

Use of motorised buggies to transport players to the side of the pitch is acceptable, as long as the patient has full cervical spine protection when needed

General trauma rules

1 Do not waste time obtaining intravenous access at the scene. A patient with hypovolaemia needs hospital transfer immediately, and cannulation can be attempted en route.
2 Do not administer intravenous fluid automatically. If the patient has a radial pulse (systolic blood pressure of at least 80 mm Hg) then the blood pressure is sufficient to perfuse the vital organs. This concept is termed *hypotensive resuscitation.*
3 Do administer high flow oxygen to all seriously injured patients. Supplementary oxygen is essential to prevent secondary spinal and brain injury.
4 Do cover wounds and apply direct pressure to obvious areas of bleeding.
5 Do administer parenteral analgesia when needed. This will lower the patient's anxiety level and subsequently reduce oxygen requirements.

after analgesia has been administered, as long as it does not delay hospital transfer.

Wounds

Methods of primary wound closure include tissue adhesive, steristrips and sutures. Care should be taken when administering tissue adhesive around the eye region, as inadvertent closure of the eyelids can result. Steristrips are useful for closing a wound quickly, although they often will come off when the player starts to sweat again. Suturing remains the most secure form of wound closure but is time consuming and needs specific skills. The combination of sutures with overlying glue is very effective, especially for head injuries. If a player has a wound closed but then does not attend an emergency department for further treatment, the pitchside medic must enquire about current tetanus immunisation status.

Soft tissue injuries

Ice and elevation are the immediate priorities, the former slows down the onset of inflammation and the latter encourages venous return and decreases dependant oedema. A non-steroidal anti-inflammatory drug works well in conjunction with paracetamol, providing the patient with analgesic and anti-inflammatory treatment.

Various devices provide good compression, although care must be taken not to bandage a limb so tightly that acute compartment syndrome develops.

Medical emergencies

Obviously, any medical emergency may occur on the field of play. With young fit athletes, however, the two most commonly encountered are acute anaphylaxis and acute asthma.

Acute anaphylaxis

Also known as immediate or type 1 hypersensitivity, this condition, which is mediated by immunoglobulin E, rapidly can be fatal because of airway compromise or cardiovascular collapse. When a susceptible athlete comes into contact with the allergen, massive histamine release occurs from mast cells bound by immunoglobulin E.

Epinephrine 500 µg should be administered intramuscularly as soon as possible and repeated after five minutes if needed. Patients with a known hypersensitivity may possess an epinephrine pen, which delivers a standard dose of 300 µg epinephrine. All patients who receive epinephrine should be transferred to hospital for further treatment, as a late phase reaction can occur some time after the initial episode.

Acute asthma

Most medical practitioners should be familiar with the treatment of this condition. Nebulised β_2 agonists and ipratropium bromide remain the first line drugs of choice for athletes who have failed to gain relief from their own inhalers. The oxygen driven nebulisers favoured by paramedic crews are able to nebulise bronchodilators more effectively than battery driven nebulisers, and any athlete with an attack of acute severe asthma should be transferred to hospital by ambulance.

The photographs of the paramedic crew, motorised buggy and ice pack on a soft tissue injury are all courtesy of Getty Images Ltd. The algorithm showing diagnosis and treatment of a tension pneumothorax is adapted from the Resuscitation and Emergency Management Onfield course manual (www.remosports.com). The photograph of the patient on a spinal board is reproduced from Grundy D, Swain A, eds. *ABC of spinal cord injury*. Oxford: Blackwell Publishing, 2002.

If a full course of three active tetanus immunisation injections has been previously administered, a booster is required every 10 years

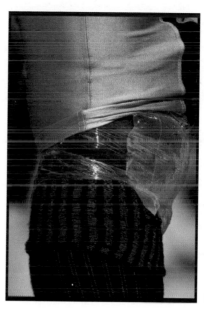

Ice on a soft tissue injury

Principles of treatment for soft tissue injuries

- Protection
- Rest
- Ice
- Elevation
- Compression
- Drugs

Antihistamine and corticosteroid drugs are only adjuncts to treatment of acute anaphylaxis and are no substitute for epinephrine

Symptoms and signs of anaphylactic shock

- Facial swelling
- Swelling of tongue and soft palate
- Stridor
- Wheeze
- Urticarial rash
- Diarrhoea
- Tachycardia
- Hypotension

3 Head injuries in sport

Paul McCrory

In sport medicine, doctors must be able to recognise and manage a spectrum of brain injury. Fortunately, serious brain injury is rare in sport (outside motor sports) and most head injuries seen are mild in nature.

Epidemiology

Traumatic brain injury is one of the leading causes of morbidity and mortality worldwide. The crude incidence for all traumatic brain injuries is estimated at about 300 per 100 000 per year, although this varies from country to country.

In hospital based surveys of brain trauma, sporting injuries contribute approximately 10-15% of all cases. Interestingly, the sports most commonly associated with severe brain injuries are golf, horse riding, and mountain climbing. Sporting related deaths because of brain injury are rare, although these have not been studied rigorously outside professional horse racing and American and Australian football.

Eighty per cent of all cases of sport related traumatic brain injuries are mild, so this group constitutes the greatest management problem for a team physician. Concussion, which is a subset of mild brain injury, needs accurate diagnosis and management to avoid long term problems.

Classification of head injury

The most widely accepted and validated method of classifying the spectrum of brain injury is the Glasgow coma scale. This scale uses eye opening, verbal response, and motor response to standard stimuli. These responses are measured six hours after injury after any resuscitation has been completed. The score is then used to separate the categories of injury severity. A score of 13-15 is designated as a mild injury, 8-12 as a moderate injury, and <8 as a severe injury.

The Glasgow coma scale also may be used for serial measurement of head injury status, where an immediate score is obtained during initial assessment of an injured patient and then performed serially to monitor progress.

Although the Glasgow coma scale is extremely useful for measuring moderate to severe traumatic brain injury, its usefulness is limited in the assessment of mild brain injury. In sports, most concussive injuries have recovered from their acute symptoms within six hours and as a result are unable to be classified under this scale. This group provides sports medicine practitioners with the greatest management dilemmas in terms of return to play decisions. Alternative classification systems have been proposed to assess concussive injuries; however, none of these have been validated scientifically.

Pathophysiology

Non-penetrating brain injury (or closed head injury) may be divided into primary and secondary injuries. Primary injury is the result of mechanical forces producing tissue deformation at the moment of injury. These deformations may result in either functional disturbance or structural disruption of cell membranes. The injury may also set off a complex cascade of biochemical, immunological, or coagulopathic changes that may further compromise cell integrity. Secondary damage occurs as a complication of primary injury.

> All people involved in the care of athletes need to have a thorough understanding of the early management of concussed athletes and the potential sequelae of such injuries that may impact upon the athletes' ability to return to sport

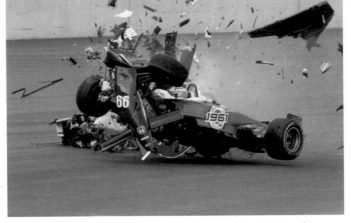

Men are more than twice as likely to have a traumatic brain injury than women, with a peak incidence among those aged 15-24 years; the most common cause of these injuries is motor vehicle crashes[1]

Glasgow coma scale

Category	Response	Score
Eye opening response (E)	Spontaneous	4
	To speech	3
	To pain	2
	No response	1
Verbal response (V)	Oriented	5
	Confused, disorientated	4
	Inappropriate words	3
	Incomprehensible sounds	2
	No response	1
Motor response (M)	Obeys commands	6
	Localises	5
	Withdraws (flexion)	4
	Abnormal flexion (posturing)	3
	Extension (posturing)	2
	No response	1

Score = E + M + V (maximum 15)

Secondary damage*

Hypoxic and ischaemic damage
Brain swelling
Hydrocephalus
Infection

*Hovda D et al. *J Neurotrauma* 1995;12:903-6

> Concussive injury by definition has no macroscopic neuropathological damage and it is speculated that the critical physiological change occurs at the cell membrane level. Recent evidence also indicates a substantial genetic basis to the outcomes in people with head injuries[2]

Specific injuries

Most texts tend to focus on neurosurgical head injuries, but >95% of brain injuries seen by sports physicians and trainers are concussive injuries. In some sports, such as motor racing, more severe brain injuries occur more often, but this chapter focuses on the commonplace injuries and their management.

Concussion

More than 35 years ago, the Committee on Head Injury Nomenclature of the US Congress of Neurological Surgeons proposed a "consensus" definition of concussion. This definition was recognised as having a number of limitations, including being unable to account for the relatively minor impact injuries that result in persistent physical or cognitive symptoms, or both. Partly in response to such issues, the First World Conference on Concussion in Sport was held in Vienna in 2002. At that meeting, a consensus definition was agreed and has now become the accepted definition of this condition.[3]

The classification of severity of concussive injury is a contentious area. At least 35 different injury severity grading systems have been published, but none has been validated scientifically. The Vienna Expert Consensus Group recommended that no specific scale be used and that all management of concussive injuries should measure individual recovery to determine return to play rather than using anecdotal grading systems and arbitrary exclusion periods.[3]

The practical management of concussion can be divided into three broad areas: immediate, early and late management. In each, the issues and treatment priorities differ considerably.

Immediate management

This is where the medic is in attendance at a sporting event and is called on to manage acute brain injury. The major priorities at this early stage are the basic principles of first aid. Once the basic aspects of care have been achieved and the patient is stabilised, consideration of removal of the patient from the field to an appropriate facility is needed. At this time, careful assessment for the presence of a cervical spine injury or other injury is needed. If an alert patient complains of neck pain, has evidence of neck tenderness or deformity, or has neurological signs indicating a spinal injury, then neck bracing and transport on a suitable spinal frame is required. If the patient is unconscious, cervical spinal cord injury should be assumed until proven otherwise. Airway protection takes precedence over any potential spinal injury. In this situation, removal of helmets or other head protectors should be performed only by individuals trained in this aspect of trauma management.

The clinical management may involve the treatment of disorientated, confused, unconscious, uncooperative, or convulsing patients. The immediate treatment priorities remain the basic first aid principles of "ABC—airway, breathing, and circulation." Once this has been established and the patient is stabilised, a full medical and neurological assessment examination should follow. On site doctors are in an ideal position to initiate the critical early steps of medical care to ensure optimal recovery from a head injury.

Early management

This refers to the situation when an athlete is brought to the medical room for assessment or to an emergency department or medical facility after the injury. Assessment of injury severity is best performed in a quiet medical room rather than the field of play. This assessment should be performed by a medical practitioner. If no doctor is available for this assessment, the athlete should be referred to a suitable facility (for example, a hospital emergency department).

Vienna expert consensus definition of concussion

Concussion is defined as "a complex pathophysiological process affecting the brain, induced by traumatic biomechanical forces." Several common features that incorporate clinical, pathological, and biomechanical injury constructs and may be used to define the nature of a concussive head injury including:

- Concussion may be caused by a direct blow to the head, face, neck, or elsewhere on the body with an "impulsive" force transmitted to the head.
- Concussion typically results in rapid onset of short lived impairment of neurological function that resolves spontaneously.
- Concussion may result in neuropathological changes, but the acute clinical symptoms largely reflect a functional disturbance rather than structural injury.
- Concussion results in a graded set of clinical syndromes that may or may not involve loss of consciousness. Resolution of the clinical and cognitive symptoms typically follows a sequential course.
- Concussion typically is associated with grossly normal structural neuroimaging studies

---

Initial on field assessment of concussion

D—Danger: ensure no immediate environmental dangers that may potentially injure the patient or treatment team. This may involve stopping play in a football match or marshalling cars on a motor racetrack.

R—Response: is the patient conscious? Can they talk?

A—Airway: ensure a clear and unobstructed airway. Remove any mouthguard or dental device that may be present.

B—Breathing: ensure patient is breathing adequately.

C—Circulation: ensure adequate circulation.

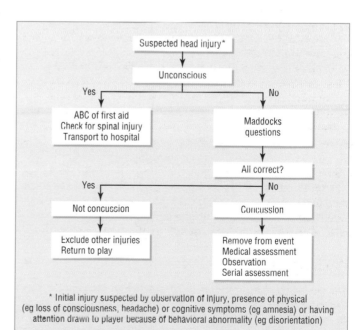

* Initial injury suspected by observation of injury, presence of physical (eg loss of consciousness, headache) or cognitive symptoms (eg amnesia) or having attention drawn to player because of behavioral abnormality (eg disorientation)

Acute concussion management

When an acutely concussed player is assessed, various aspects of the history and examination are important. The common symptoms of concussion have been examined in prospective studies and include headache, dizziness, blurred vision, and nausea. The presence of headache is not confined to concussion, however, with up to 50% of sporting athletes reporting exercise related headache. As much emphasis is placed on headache as an important symptom of concussion, medical assessment needs to be accurate in ascertaining the nature and cause of the player's symptoms.

Also important to note is that neither the presence nor duration of loss of consciousness is a critical aspect of concussion assessment. Numerous studies have shown that loss of consciousness is not prognostic in this setting, and, accordingly, injury classification and management algorithms should not be based on this symptom.

A full neurological examination is important when a concussed athlete is examined. The major management priorities at this stage are to establish an accurate diagnosis and exclude a catastrophic intracranial injury, so this part of the examination should be particularly thorough.

Recently, simple neuropsychological tests have created considerable interest as a means of objectively assessing concussed athletes. The standard approach of asking the orientation items (for example, day, date, year, time, date of birth, and so on) has been shown to be unreliable after concussive injury. This aspect of memory remains relatively intact in the face of concussive injury and should not be used. More useful, as demonstrated in prospective studies, are questions of recent memory.[4] A typical question battery is rapid to administer and validated scientifically in making a diagnosis of concussion. Alternative systems have been proposed, but these are lengthier to administer and not suited to most sports.[5]

Although a trainer or non-medical person may use the Maddocks questions, or other similar tools, to diagnose concussion (or suspect the diagnosis), all concussed athletes should be referred for urgent medical assessment. Most high level amateur and professional teams in fact will have their own medical staff to make the diagnosis; however, where teams lack this facility, concussed athletes need to be referred to a local medical provider or hospital emergency department to undergo a full assessment.

When the presence of a concussive injury is determined, the patient needs to be monitored serially until full recovery ensues. If the concussed player is discharged home after recovery, they should be in the care of a responsible adult. The author's policy is to give the patient and their attendant a head injury advice card upon discharge.

The treating doctor also must decide who should be referred to a hospital emergency facility or neurosurgical centre. A number of urgent indications exist. Apart from these "cookbook" type approaches, referral to such a centre depends on the experience, ability, and competency of the doctor at hand. The overall approach should be "when in doubt, refer."

Late management and return to play
This refers to when a player has sustained a concussive injury previously and now is presenting for advice or clearance before resuming sport. The main management priorities at this stage are assessment of recovery and application of the appropriate return to sport guidelines. Any clearance to return to sport is the province of a medical practitioner, ideally with experience of these sporting injuries, and it should not be undertaken by non-medical personnel.

Criteria for return to sport after a concussion remain the most contentious area of debate. Although the traditional

---

Early assessment of concussion—history
- Time and place of injury
- Mechanism of injury (eyewitness or video)
- Presence or duration of loss of consciousness
- Behaviour after injury
- Presence of convulsions post-injury
- Past medical history
- Drug use

Post concussion memory assessment (Maddocks questions)
- Which ground are we at?
- Which team are we playing today?
- Who is your opponent at present?
- Which quarter is it?
- How far into the quarter is it?
- Which side scored the last goal?
- Which team did we play last week?
- Did we win last week?

Head injury advice

This patient has received an injury to the head. A careful medical examination has been carried out, and no sign of any serious complications has been found.

Recovery is expected to be rapid, but in such cases to be quite certain is not possible.

If you notice any change in behaviour, vomiting, dizziness, headache, double vision, or excessive drowsiness, please telephone _____ or the nearest hospital emergency department immediately.

Other important points:
- No alcohol
- No analgesics or pain killers
- No driving

Patient's name: _____
Date and time of injury: _____
Date of medical review: _____
Treating doctor: _____

Clinic telephone number _____

Indications for urgent referral
- Fractured skull
- Penetrating skull trauma
- Deterioration in conscious state after injury
- Focal neurological signs
- Confusion or impairment of consciousness >30 minutes
- Loss of consciousness >5 minutes
- Persistent vomiting or increasing headache post injury
- Any convulsive movements
- More than one episode of concussive injury in a session
- Where assessment is difficult (for example, in an intoxicated patient)
- Children with head injuries
- High risk patients (for example, haemophilia or anticoagulant use)
- Inadequate post injury supervision
- High risk injury mechanism (for example, high velocity impact)

approach is to advocate a mandatory arbitrary exclusion period from sport, this strategy has been rejected by the Vienna Expert Consensus Group.[3] Use of individualised neuropsychological testing in conjunction with clinical assessment currently is the recommended basis for return to play. Where any doubt exists, clinical judgment should prevail.

Neuropsychological testing to determine recovery and guide return to play is increasingly accepted worldwide. In Australian and American football, such strategies have been used since 1985. More recently, professional horse racing, ice hockey, and a number of other sports have followed similar strategies. Post-injury tests usually are compared with a player's baseline or preseason performance. The most important conceptual point is the understanding that these tests are not designed to be used as a diagnostic test for concussion in acute situations. In practice, the test battery is performed once all post-concussive symptoms have resolved, as a means of objectively measuring return to baseline level of function. Although these are not yet in widespread use, they may provide a simple aid for medical practitioners to objectively measure recovery from concussion.

Specific post-concussion risks
Second impact syndrome—Diffuse cerebral oedema is a rare but well recognised complication of mild traumatic brain injury in sport that occurs predominantly in children and teenagers. The impact, however trivial, sets in train the rapid development of cerebral swelling that usually results in brainstem herniation and death. Its cause is unknown, but it is thought to involve disordered cerebral vascular autoregulation.

Concussive or impact convulsions—Concussive convulsions in collision sport are an uncommon but dramatic association with minor head injury. They are thought to represent a reflex phenomenon and are not associated with structural brain injury. From a clinical standpoint, late seizures do not occur, antiepileptic therapy is not indicated, and prohibition from collision sport is unwarranted. The treating doctor can reassure the patient that concussive convulsions are benign, and the overall management should centre on appropriate treatment of the concussive injury itself.

Prevention of concussion
Concussive brain injury may be minimised in sport by relatively few methods. The brain is not an organ that can be conditioned to withstand injury. Thus, extrinsic mechanisms of injury prevention must be sought.

Helmets have been proposed as a means of protecting the head and theoretically reducing the risk of brain injury. In sports in which there are high speed collisions or that have the potential for missile injuries (for example, in baseball) or falls onto hard surfaces, published evidence shows the effectiveness of sport specific helmets in reducing head injuries, particularly skull fractures.[2] For other sports, such as football and rugby, no sport specific helmet has been shown to be of proven benefit in reducing rates of head injury. Some believe that the use of protective equipment may alter playing behaviour deleteriously, so that the athlete actually has an increased risk of brain injury. This is particularly an issue with children and adolescents who may adopt risk taking behaviour when wearing protective equipment.

Although the use of correctly fitting mouth guards can reduce the rate of dental, orofacial and mandibular injuries, evidence that they reduce cerebral injuries largely is theoretical. Clinical evidence for a beneficial effect in reducing concussion rates has not been shown scientifically.[2]

Guiding policy for return to sport

- Until **completely** symptom free, concussed athletes should not resume any training or competition
- This should be assessed initially at rest and then after a provocative exercise challenge
- This is recommended to be aerobic exercise, and the athlete should exercise until their heart rate reaches 80% maximum predicted heart rate
- Once the acute concussive symptoms resolve at rest and exercise, a graduated plan of return to low level aerobic training, followed by non-contact drills and finally contact play will allow close monitoring of the development of any adverse symptoms
- Persisting or newly developing symptoms need further follow up and detailed medical evaluation

---

Although repeated concussive injuries have been proposed as the basis for second impact syndrome, the evidence is not compelling. More likely is that a single impact of any severity may result in this rare complication, but that participation in sport draws attention to incidental concussive injuries

---

In players who have concussive convulsions, the universally good outcome and absence of structural injury or long term neuropsychological damage reflects the benign nature of these episodes

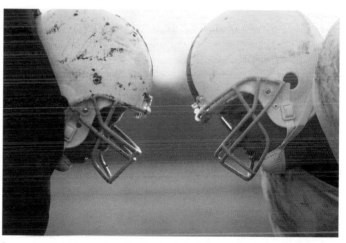

In sports (such as American football) where there are high speed collisions or falls onto hard surfaces, sport specific helmets can reduce the number of head injuries

---

Possible methods for preventing concussion

- Helmets
- Mouth guards
- Rule changes and enforcement
- Neck muscle conditioning

Consideration of rule changes (for example, no head checking in ice hockey) and rule enforcement to reduce the head injury rate may be appropriate when a clear cut mechanism is implicated in a particular sport. For most sports, however, head injuries are an accidental by product of normal play, so rule changes and rule enforcement have little effect on rates of head injuries. Nevertheless, the promotion of fair play and respect for opponents are ethical values that should be encouraged in all sports and by sporting associations.

Neck muscle conditioning may be of value in reducing impact forces transmitted to the brain. Biomechanical concepts dictate that the energy from an impacting object is dispersed over the greater mass of an athlete if the head is held rigidly. Although attractive from a theoretical standpoint, little scientific evidence shows the effectiveness of such measures.

Traumatic intracerebral haematoma and contusion

Traumatic intracerebral haematomas are divided into acute and delayed types. Clinical signs and symptoms depend on the size and location of the intracerebral haematoma, as well as the speed of development. In most cases, at least a brief period of confusion or loss of consciousness is reported. Only one third of patients remain lucid throughout their course. Overall cognitive impairment and the speed and quality of recovery are related strongly to coexistent cerebral injury. An intracerebral haematoma that occurs in isolation with a volume <30 ml is compatible with a favourable recovery. Overall, death rates are in the range of 25% to 30%. Medical management of intracerebral haematomas is directed primarily at reducing post-traumatic oedema and cerebral ischaemia.

Subdural haematoma

Subdural haematomas can be the result of non-penetrating or penetrating trauma to the head. In both cases, extravasation of blood into the subdural space is the mechanism for haematoma formation because of stretching and subsequent rupture of bridging cerebral veins. These injuries are typically seen after falls onto hard surfaces or assaults with non-deformable objects rather than low velocity injuries. Clinical signs and symptoms depend on the size and location of the subdural haematoma, as well as the speed of development. In most cases, at least a brief period of confusion or loss of consciousness is reported. Soft tissue injuries usually are seen at the site of impact. Enlargement of the haematoma, or an increase in oedema surrounding it, produces an additional mass effect. Often, the impact produces a coexisting severe brain injury that explains, in large part, the poor outcome of acute subdural haematoma.

Extradural haematoma

Irrespective of the nature of inciting trauma, a direct blow to the head is essential for extradural haematoma formation. As the skull is deformed by the impact and the adherent dura forcefully detached, haemorrhage may occur into the preformed extradural space. The source of bleeding may be arterial or venous, or both. Haemorrhage from a fracture line may also accumulate to create a mass lesion in the extradural space. The expanding extradural lesion only partially accounts for the neurological morbidity observed with extradural haematomas. Coincident intradural pathology is encountered in up to 50% of cases. In general, sequelae of these lesions dictate the degree of residual functional impairment in patients who survive extradural haematoma. The clinical variability associated with extradural haemorrhage is remarkable. Rarely, extradural haematomas may be asymptomatic; most, however, present with non-specific signs and symptoms referable to an intracranial mass lesion. Alteration in consciousness is a

> Education of players, parents, coaches, and other staff plays an important part in ensuring that fair play and respect for opponents are implemented on the field of play

---

Traumatic intracerebral haematoma

- Acute—occur at the time of the initial head injury
- Delayed—reported to occur as early as six hours after injury to as long as several weeks

---

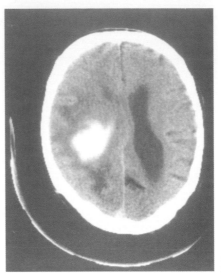

Computed tomogram of intracranial bleed

Signs of substantial head trauma that can result in subdural haematomas

- Periorbital and postauricular ecchymoses
- Haemotympanum
- Cerebrospinal fluid otorrhoea or rhinorrhoea
- Facial fractures

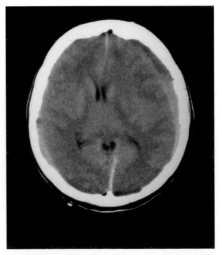

Computed tomogram of subdural haematoma

> In the supratentorial compartment, haemorrhage from the middle meningeal artery contributes to at least 50% of extradural haematomas; bleeding from the middle meningeal veins accounts for an additional 33%

hallmark manifestation of extradural haematoma. The so-called "lucid interval" occurs in less than one third of patients, and is not a sensitive diagnostic discriminator. The natural course of large traumatic extradural haematomas is dismal if the lesion is unrecognised or untreated. In most cases, the expanding mass lesion precipitates progressive neurological dysfunction. Rapid diagnosis and prompt surgical evacuation afford the best chance for optimising outcome.

Traumatic subarachnoid haemorrhage

Traumatic subarachnoid haemorrhage usually is a consequence of vertebral artery injury—a tear or dissection—although it also may be due to tearing of meningeal vessels. Subarachnoid bleeding typically presents with florid meningeal symptoms such as headache, neck stiffness, and photophobia. The most common initial symptoms in vertebral artery injury are neck pain and occipital headache that may precede the onset of neurological symptoms from a few seconds to several weeks Headache symptoms have been noted in most cases to be ipsilateral to the vascular injury and the pain usually radiates to the temporal region, frontal area, eye, or ear. None of the reported cases had cervical tenderness or objective restriction of neck movement, although subjective exacerbation of pain did occur with neck movement. The outcome of such injuries often is poor

Diffuse cerebral oedema

The injured brain has long been known to swell in the cranial cavity. The increase in intracerebral volume—whatever its cause or nature—eventually will be associated with an increase in intracranial pressure. In the first few hours and days after a severe head injury, intracranial pressure often is raised because of alterations in the volume of the cerebrovascular bed, whereas brain swelling after this time is because of an increase in water content of the brain tissue. Downward displacement of the cerebrum because of increased intracranial pressure results in compression of the midbrain through the tentorial notch or coning. Treatment for elevated intracranial pressure because of oedema relies on several methods; however, the outcome generally is poor and reflects the initiating cause of the oedema, as well as the variable response to treatment

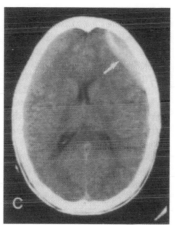

Computed tomogram of an acute extradural heamatoma

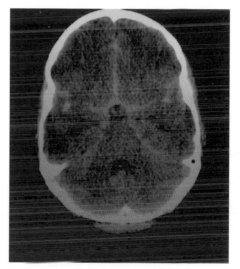

Computed tomogram of a subarachnoid haemorrhage

Management of traumatic brain injury

Acute management

The management of an acute brain injury largely follows the approach for concussion. The so-called primary and secondary survey of injuries, although popular in the literature about trauma, does not reflect current practice in sports medicine.

Vital signs must be recorded after an injury. Abnormalities may reflect brain stem dysfunction. Although head injury produces several types of respiratory patterns, an acute rise in intracranial pressure with central herniation usually manifests rising blood pressure and falling pulse rate (the Cushing response). Hypotension rarely is because of brain injury, except as a terminal event, and alternate sources for the drop in blood pressure should be aggressively sought and treated. This point cannot be underestimated, as cerebral hypotension and hypoxia are the main determinants of outcome after brain injury and are easily treatable.

A neurological examination should be performed, including measurement of the score on the Glasgow coma scale. Findings of this examination must be recorded, so that an overall trend in improving or deteriorating mental function can be documented clearly and objectively. In addition, palpation of the skull, which is quick and simple, should be a component of every physical examination in patients with head trauma.

Anecdotal evidence shows that massive traumatic cerebral oedema, documented by computed tomography, occurs within 20 minutes of cerebral injury

The history of the injury often gives important clues to its nature. This often needs an eyewitness account; in the case of professional sport, videotape analysis may be available

The importance of the initial neurological examination is that it serves as a reference against which other serial neurological examinations may be compared

When time permits, a more thorough physical examination should be performed to exclude coexistent injuries or detect signs of skull injury. Restlessness is a frequent accompaniment of brain injury or cerebral hypoxia, and it may be confused with a belligerent patient who is presumably intoxicated. If the patient is unconscious but restless, attention should be given to the possibility of increased cerebral hypoxia, a distended bladder, painful wounds, or tight casts. Only these are definitely ruled out should drug treatment be considered.

Investigations in head trauma

A number of indications exist for emergent cranial computed tomography in the initial evaluation of patients with head injuries. Evaluation by computed tomography should start as soon as the patient is haemodynamically stable and once immediately life threatening injuries have been dealt with. As the incidence of delayed formation of extradural haematoma after head trauma is substantial, any deterioration in the neurological examination warrants prompt evaluation by computed tomography, even if a previous study was normal.

The role of magnetic resonance imaging in the evaluation of acute head trauma is limited. Compared with computed tomography, magnetic resonance imaging is time consuming, expensive, and less sensitive to acute haemorrhage and associated bony injury. Moreover, access to critically ill patients is restricted during lengthy periods of image acquisition, and the strong magnetic fields generated by the scanner need the use of non-ferromagnetic resuscitative equipment.

In the initial assessment of patients with head injuries, other more traditional diagnostic tools have largely been supplanted by computed tomography of the cranium. Plain skull radiographs are inexpensive and easily obtained, and often demonstrate fractures in patients with extradural haemorrhage. However, the predictive value of such films is poor, as one finding is not requisite for the other. Lateral shift of the pineal gland, indicative of hemispheric mass effect, is a non-specific and highly variable finding.

Management of acute post-traumatic seizures

As described previously, impact seizures or concussive convulsions are rare but well recognised sequelae of head impacts. These occur within seconds of injury, are not epileptic, and require no specific management beyond the treatment of the underlying concussive injury.

In contrast, post-traumatic epilepsy may occur and is more common as the severity of brain injury increases. A convulsing patient is at increased risk of hypoxia, with resultant exacerbation of the underlying brain injury. Maintenance of cerebral oxygenation and perfusion pressure (blood pressure) is critical in the management of such patients.

Non-brain head injury

As well as the various brain injuries described above, sports doctors should be familiar with the various soft tissue, bony, ocular, and other injuries that may occur to the head. Soft tissue injuries (such as contusions) and sense organ injuries (such as eye injuries) are discussed in chapters 5 and 6.

Scalp wounds, although dramatic in appearance, usually heal well if good wound management is followed. Blood loss from scalp wounds may be extensive, particularly in children, but it rarely causes shock. In the case of severed large vessels (for example, superficial temporal artery), the arterial bleeder should be located, clamped, and ligated. The wound always should be inspected carefully and inside the laceration should

---

Indications for emergent neuroimaging

- History of loss of consciousness
- Depressed level of consciousness
- Focal neurological deficit
- Deteriorating neurological status
- Skull fracture
- Progressive or severe headache
- Persistent nausea or vomiting
- Post-traumatic seizure
- Mechanism of injury that suggests high risk of intracranial haemorrhage
- Examination obscured by alcohol, drugs, metabolic derangement, or post-ictal state
- Patient inaccessibility for serial neurological examinations
- Coagulopathy and other high risk medical conditions

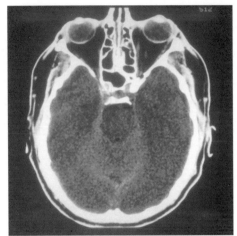

Computed tomogram showing brain swelling

Magnetic resonance imaging is best suited to defining associated parenchymal injuries after the acute event

Drugs used to treat post-traumatic epilepsy

- Intravenous phenytoin (or fosphenytoin) usually is the drug of choice in this situation, because a loading dose can be administered intravenously to rapidly achieve therapeutic concentrations and because phenytoin does not impair consciousness
- Benzodiazepines (such as lorazepam and clonazepam) can be used for acute treatment of post-traumatic seizures, but they will produce at least transient impairment of consciousness
- Phenytoin, none of the benzodiazepines, and no other antiepileptic drug has been shown to be effective for preventing development of post-traumatic epilepsy

be palpated with a sterile glove for signs of an underlying skull fracture. All cases that involve open fractures or depressed skull fractures should have a neurosurgical consultation. The wound should be irrigated with copious amounts of saline before it is closed. Any debris, including hair, must be removed from the wound. Primary repair should be accomplished with the use of a sterile technique.

The scalp and soft tissues of the head and neck are extremely well vascularised, and this often results in copious bleeding if these structures are injured. The doctor should adopt universal precautions against blood borne infections such as hepatitis B virus, hepatitis C virus, and HIV.

Summary

Traumatic head injury represents one of the most common types of injury in sporting situations. Although most such injuries are mild concussions that recover without long term sequelae, the potential exists for more severe brain injury that may have a catastrophic outcome. Sports medicine doctors should be familiar with the clinical signs and symptoms of such injuries and have a clear, well practiced management algorithm.

The photograph of the racing car crash is courtesy of Getty Images.

Further reading
- Jennett B, Bond M. Assessment of outcome after severe brain damage: a practical scale. *Lancet* 1975;1:480-4
- Hovda D, Lee S, Smith M, von Stuck S, Bergschneider M, Kelly D, et al. The neurochemical and metabolic cascade following brain injury: moving from animal models to man. *J Neurotrauma* 1995;12:903-6
- McCrory PR, Berkovic SF. Second impact syndrome. *Neurology* 1998;50:677-83
- McCrory PR, Bladin PF, Berkovic SF. Retrospective study of concussive convulsions in elite Australian rules and rugby league footballers: phenomenology, aetiology, and outcome. *BMJ* 1997;314:171-4
- Finch C, McIntosh A, McCrory P. What do under 15 year old schoolboy rugby union players think about protective headgear? *Br J Sports Med* 2001;35:89-95

1 Jennett B. Epidemiology of head injury. *J Neurol Neurosurg Psych* 1996;60:362-9.
2 Johnston K, McCrory P, Mohtadi N, Meeuwisse W. Evidence based review of sport-related concussion—clinical science. *Clin J Sport Med* 2001;11:150-60
3 Aubry M, Cantu R, Dvorak J, Graf-Baumann T, Johnston K, Kelly J et al. Summary and agreement statement of the first International Conference on Concussion in Sport, Vienna 2001. *Br J Sports Med* 2002;36:6-10.
4 Maddocks DL, Dicker GD, Saling MM. The assessment of orientation following concussion in athletes. *Clin J Sport Med* 1995;5:32-5.
5 McCrea M, Kelly J, Randolph C, Kluge J, Bartolic E, Finn G et al. Standardised assessment of concussion (SAC): On site mental status evaluation of the athlete. *J Head Trauma Rehab* 1998;13:27-36.

4 Injury to face and jaw

K R Postlethwaite

Although interpersonal violence is the most common cause of facial injury, sports, especially the contact sports, also are often associated with facial injury. Recent studies have shown that the incidence is increasing.

The type of facial injury that can occur during sporting activities varies from simple cuts and abrasions or minor dental injury to severely comminuted facial fractures. The latter may be associated with head and cervical spine injury. Initial attention should focus on the airway and the control of bleeding.

Injuries received often relate to the mechanism of injury, and a good history from the patient or witnesses is important for guiding clinical examination. Accurate diagnosis will aid effective initial treatment and appropriate specialist referral.

Soft tissue injuries

Abrasions
Contaminated simple abrasions need thorough cleaning and debridement to prevent infection and ugly pigmentation. This latter occurs most commonly when the abrasion is because of contact with a tarmacadam surface. Although simple debridement of superficial abrasions is possible, when large areas are involved or where there is gross contamination, treatment may need local or sometimes general anaesthesia. Antibiotic prescription also should be considered.

Haematomas
Haematomas often settle spontaneously and rarely need drainage. Blunt injury to the ear, however, may result in a subperichondrial haematoma, which can result in cartilage deformity (cauliflower ear). Such haematomas should be drained by needle aspiration or a small incision, and a pressure dressing should be applied carefully. Nasal septal haematomas again need evacuation to prevent necrosis of the underlying cartilage. Very occasionally, large haematomas undergo liquefaction and exhibit fluctuance. If they fail to absorb after 7-10 days, drainage can be helpful.

Lacerations
Lacerations should be debrided thoroughly, and antibiotics prescribed when gross contamination has occurred. Thought also should be given to the need for tetanus prophylaxis. When lacerations are small, superficial, and in uncomplicated areas of the face, accurate suturing under local anaesthesia using fine instruments and 5/0 or 6/0 monofilament nylon is appropriate. Very superficial wounds sometimes can be treated effectively with adhesive tapes (sterile strips).

Deeper lacerations will need resorbable subcutaneous sutures, such as polyglactic acid, to approximate the skin edges before placement of skin sutures. Skin sutures can be covered in a polyantibiotic ointment (chloramphenicol or polymyxin B sulphate plus bacitracin zinc) to prevent infection and aid removal at 5-7 days.

Care should be taken with small puncture wounds. They may represent the entry point of a foreign body and so will need radiographic examination and possibly exploration.

Facial nerve function should be checked, as lacerations that involve sectioning of nerve branches should be referred urgently for microsurgical repair. Shaving the eyebrow before

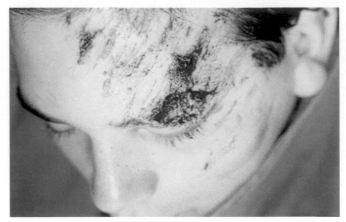
Extensive contaminated wound of forehead requiring thorough debridement and repair

Lacerations requiring specialist referral
- Lacerations involving the lip vermilion, eyelids, and lacrimal apparatus
- Be aware of nerve injuries; check facial nerve function
- Parotid duct injury
- Where there is tissue loss or full thickness laceration of the lips
- Lacerations involving the cartilage of the ear or nose
- Intraoral mucosal lacerations

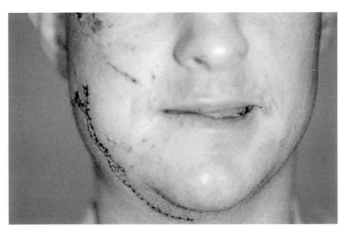
Laceration with severing of the cervical branch of the facial nerve

Systematic process for checking facial nerve function

Ask the patient to:

- Look upwards or frown (frontalis branch)
- Screw up the eyes (zygomatico-temporal)
- Twitch the nose (buccal)
- Purse the lips (mandibular and cervical)

suturing of lacerations is not recommended, as it can lead to misalignment and problems of regrowth.

Intraoral lacerations can be difficult to suture because of problems of adequate access. They are probably best referred to a maxillofacial unit.

Dental injury

Injury to the mouth may cause soft tissue injury and often can be associated with dental injury. Teeth may be fractured, mobilised, subluxed, or avulsed.

Fracturing of the teeth may involve exposure of the sensitive dentine or dental pulp, which can be extremely sensitive and painful. Fractured teeth need appropriate dressing by a dental surgeon. Mobilised teeth need splinting and thorough dental evaluation to exclude fracture of the root and monitor vitality.

Subluxation (displacement) of teeth needs repositioning, usually under local anaesthesia, and splinting for 7-10 days. Avulsed teeth may be reimplanted successfully, although inappropriate first aid will affect the prognosis adversely; success depends on correct initial treatment.

Prevention of dental injury by the use of correctly fitted mouth guards should be mandatory in all contact sports.

Maxillofacial fractures

Such injuries always should be suspected when any facial trauma has occurred. If any doubt exists, referral for specialist advice should be made. Be aware that facial fractures may be associated with head and cervical spine injury.

The facial skeleton is divided into thirds to aid systematic examination. Fractures of the nasal bones, cheekbone (zygoma), and mandible are the most common facial bony injuries that occur in sport.

A general examination of the face should be carried out; this should include a visual inspection, looking for deformity and asymmetry. This is aided by cleaning blood from the face. The facial skeleton then should be palpated, looking for areas of tenderness and possible bony steps, which are felt most commonly around the orbital margins. Areas of facial paraesthesia often indicate the presence of fractures because of damage to the various branches of the trigeminal nerve, as they pass through bony canals.

Nasal fractures

Nasal fractures may be associated with nasal bleeding that usually responds to local measures, such as application of pressure or occasionally nasal packing with ribbon gauze impregnated with petroleum jelly.

When prolonged or excessive bleeding occurs, this may indicate more extensive facial bony injury. On occasions, Foley catheters or Brighton's balloons may be needed to function as postnasal packs. When seen immediately after the injury, deformity of the nose may be apparent, but rapid onset of swelling often masks this.

Surgical treatment usually involves a closed manipulation of the fracture and application of a nasal splint. This treatment may be carried out immediately, but it is often delayed for 7-10 days to allow swelling to settle. In some instances, late surgical intervention is indicated to correct deviation of the septal cartilage that is fractured and deviated, causing blockage of the nasal airway.

Zygomatic (cheekbone) fractures

Fractures of the zygomatic bones result in flattening of the affected side and facial asymmetry that is, again, often masked

Management of avulsed teeth

- If the tooth is retrieved successfully, hold the crown, not the root, to avoid damaging the periodontal ligament remnants
- Gently wash the tooth under cold tap water and, if possible, replace in the socket and retain in this position by gently biting on a gauze or clean handkerchief
- If this is not possible, or when inhalation is possible, transport the tooth in milk or isotonic fluid if this is available
- When avulsed teeth or fragments are not accounted for and when loss of consciousness has occurred, the possibility of inhalation should be excluded by chest x ray
- Refer for further specialist treatment

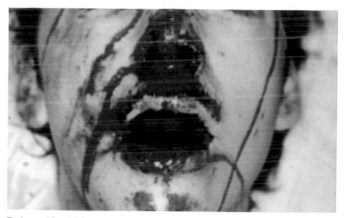

Patient with mid-face facial fractures; there was mobility of the maxilla

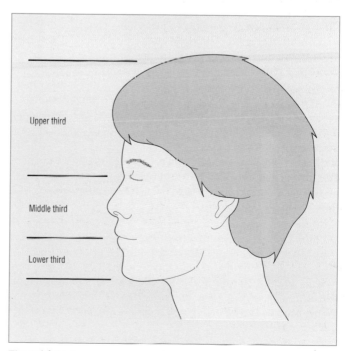

The facial thirds

by swelling. Injury to the infraorbital nerve that causes a characteristic area of facial numbness invariably occurs with fractures involving the zygomatic body.

As the zygoma forms the lateral and inferior orbital walls, associated injury often occurs to the eye and periorbital tissues. The most frequent features seen are subconjunctival echymosis, blurring of vision, and diplopia. When the zygomatic arch is fractured, mouth opening may be limited because of the depressed arch impinging on the underlying temporalis muscle at its insertion to the coronoid process of the mandible.

Radiographic evaluation is carried out with occipitomental and submentovertex views to confirm the presence of a fracture and the degree of displacement. Treatment involves open reduction and internal fixation with small bone plates.

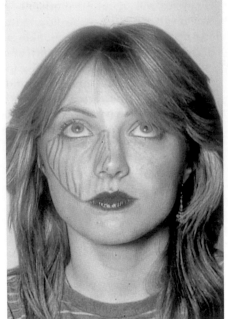

Area of numbness associated with infraorbital nerve injury

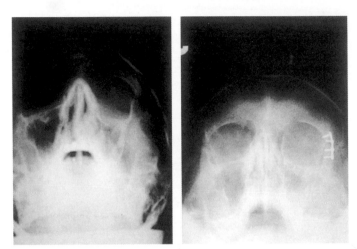

Depressed fracture of left zygoma (left) and reduction and internal fixation of fracture (right)

Internal orbital fractures

These are more commonly known as blow out fractures and usually involve the orbital floor and occasionally the medial wall. A blow out fracture should be suspected in any injury that involves a blow to the orbital area. They may be difficult to diagnose clinically and often are missed. The main features seen are diplopia, with "tethering" of the affected eye (usually to upward or lateral gaze), together with paraesthesia as a result of injury to the infraorbital nerve in its bony canal. In addition, eye movement may be painful.

A sunken appearance (enophthalmos) of the eye may be a late feature, but it often is initially masked by periorbital swelling. Investigation usually involves a computed tomography scan, which, as well as confirming the fracture, provides information as to the site and extent of the defect.

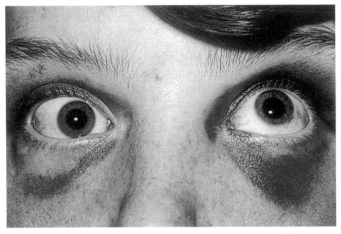

Diplopia—tethering of the right eye to upward gaze indicates a blow out fracture

Treatment

All cases should undergo maxillofacial and ophthalmic assessment before treatment, which may involve freeing of the trapped tissue and repair of the defect to restore the contour of the orbit.

Mandibular fractures

The mandible is a horseshoe-shaped bone and fractures often occur bilaterally. They also occur at points of weakness, the condylar neck being the most common site.

Pain and difficulty in occluding the teeth are an indication of mandibular fracture. Due to damage to the mandibular nerve within its bony canal, paraesthesia of the lower lip on the affected side is often seen.

Bony steps are not easily palpable extra-orally apart from grossly displaced fractures. However, intraoral examination may

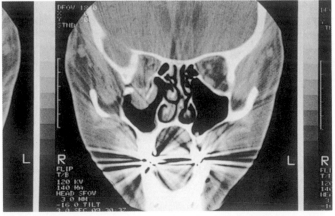

Coronal computed tomography scan confirms a blow out fracture of the right orbital floor with prolapse of tissue from the orbit into the underlying maxillary sinus

be more helpful in revealing obvious steps in the lower dental arch or a deranged bite, together with mucosal bruising and lacerations.

Treatment usually involves open reduction and internal fixation with small plates applied to the bone surface, most commonly via an intraoral approach.

Fractures of the middle third of face

Middle third facial fractures are usually seen following high velocity injuries or, on occasions, particularly violent assaults, they are not commonly seen following sporting injury, but nonetheless should always be considered in trauma to the face. They should be suspected especially when there is derangement of the dental occlusion, palpable bony steps, along the infra-orbital margin, facial sensory disturbance and nasal bleeding.

Middle third fractures are also associated with mobility of the maxilla which may be seen when the upper teeth are grasped and pressure applied.

The fractures may be classified using the Le Fort description. Fractures at the II or III levels may involve rhinorrhoea of the cerebrospinal fluid.

Summary

Soft tissue injury

Facial and intraoral lacerations may need specialist referral. Be aware of underlying nerve injuries—check the patient's facial nerve function.

Dental injury

If the tooth is successfully retrieved and complete, hold the crown, **not** the root, to avoid damaging the periodontal ligament remnants. Replacement in the socket as soon as possible is vital to success. If needed, transport should only be in an isotonic solution, if available, milk, or the patient's own saliva.

Facial bony injury

In all patients with facial trauma with or without considerable soft tissue injury, underlying bony injury always should be suspected, with early referral for specialist advice if in any doubt. After such an injury, the patient should avoid contact sport for 6-8 weeks.

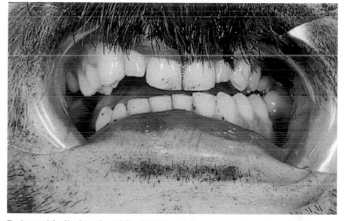

Patient with displaced middle third facial fracture and associated malocclusion (deranged bite)

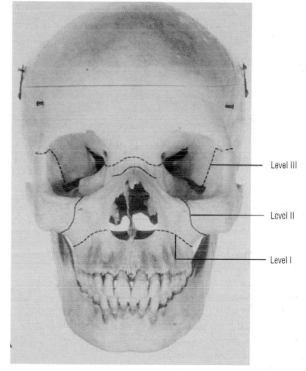

Le Fort fractures

Level III

Level II

Level I

Further reading

- Crow R. Diagnosis and management of sports-related injuries to the face. *Dental clin N Am* 1991;35:719-32
- Emshoff R, Schoning H, Rothler G, Waldhart E. Trends in the incidence and cause of sport-related mandibular fractures. *J oral maxillofac surg* 1997;55:585-92
- Rowe NL, Williams JW, eds. *Maxillofacial injuries.* Edinburgh: Churchill Livingstone, 1994

5 Eye injuries in sport

Caroline J MacEwen

Most eye injuries associated with sport are superficial and involve only the external eye or surrounding tissues. In about a third of cases, damage occurs to the intraocular structures, with potentially sight threatening consequences. Sport is responsible for 25-40% of all eye injuries that are severe enough to require hospital admission. Most of these injuries are entirely preventable.

Spectrum of injury

Superficial blunt trauma

Most sporting eye injuries are caused by balls or collisions with other players and, therefore, are blunt in nature. The most common effects of blunt trauma include:

- Periorbital contusion or "black eye". Although not a serious injury, this may cause tense eyelid swelling that prevents adequate examination of the underlying globe. To force the lids open is inadvisable and may lead to failure to identify a serious ocular injury.
- Subconjunctival haemorrhage, easily recognised as a diffuse, uniform, bright red area that covers some or all of the white of the eye, commonly occurs in association with a black eye.
- In corneal abrasion, the corneal epithelium often is disrupted or removed by a direct blow causing an acutely painful corneal abrasion.

Blow out fractures

Blow out fractures occur when the eye is struck with considerable force and the intraorbital pressure rises abruptly, so that the floor of the orbit "blows out" into the maxillary antrum. It may be accompanied by prolapse of the contents of the inferior orbital, which causes:

- Enophthalmos
- Infraorbital anaesthesia
- Double vision.

Diagnosis is clinical, but computed tomography is needed if surgery is considered necessary, usually for persistent diplopia.

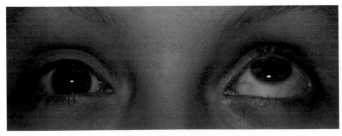

Patient unable to elevate right eye due to a blow out fracture

Intraocular blunt trauma

Severe blunt injuries may damage the intraocular contents:

- Hyphaema—the most frequent sign of severe blunt injury is hyphaema, or bleeding into the anterior chamber. This usually comes from a tear in the iris, although presence of hyphaema implies considerable intraocular trauma and that urgent specialist attention is required.

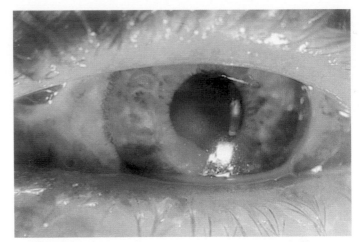

Corneal abrasion stained with fluorescein

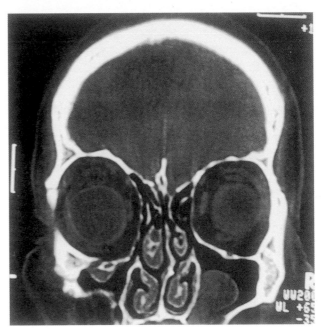

Computed tomogram showing blow out fracture of the orbital floor

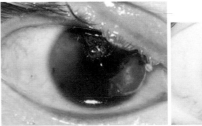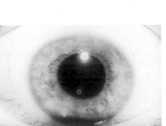

Diffuse fresh hyphaema causing a hazy appearance of the anterior segment structures (left), and level hyphaema caused by settling of blood in the anterior chamber (right)

- Retinal tear—this predisposes to a retinal detachment.
- Vitreous haemorrhage—vitreous haemorrhage is caused by damage to retinal vessels.
- Commotio retina—traumatic oedema of the sensory retina can be extensive. If the macular area is involved, it carries a poor prognosis for visual recovery.
- Choroidal ruptures—these usually occur in the macular area and lead to considerable reduction in central vision.
- Rupture of the globe—this is rare, but it may be the result of severe blunt trauma. The vision is reduced dramatically and severe subconjunctival bleeding and swelling occur.

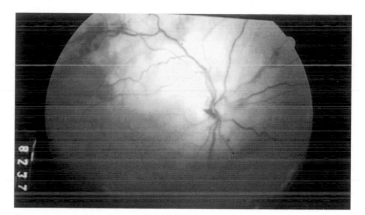

Area of commotio retina—pallor of the retina with associated haemorrhage

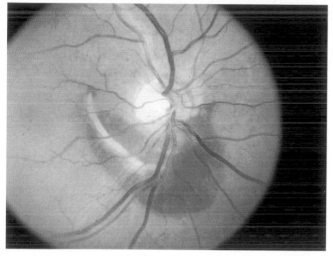

Choroidal rupture surrounded by retinal haemorrhage

Penetrating injuries

Penetrating injuries from rackets, sticks, fingers, or fish hooks entering the globe fortunately are rare. They should be suspected if the anterior chamber seems shallower on the injured side or if the pupil is irregular, as the iris plugs the wound. The extent of injury depends on how far the object has entered the eye, but multiple intraocular structures may be affected, resulting in a poor visual outcome.

Small foreign particles

Small pieces of foreign material, such as dust or grit, often are blown or flicked onto the eye during any outdoor activity. These little particles may remain on the cornea, causing intense pain. In some instances, they settle under the upper lid as subtarsal foreign bodies and rub up and down, scratching the front of the eye as it opens and closes. Foreign bodies that penetrate the eye are rare in sport.

Burns

Skiers and climbers are susceptible to "snow blindness" because of burns from ultraviolet light that cause corneal de-epithelialisation. Chemical burns are uncommon, but they can occur in swimmers as a result of excess chlorination of swimming pools and from particles of lime from pitch markings that accidentally enter the eye.

Assessment and first aid

The role of the attending doctor is to:

- Determine whether or not an eye injury is serious
- Treat any minor injuries
- Sanction return to the field if considered appropriate.

The eye should be examined in a systematic fashion with good light. Surface examination of the eye is supplemented with

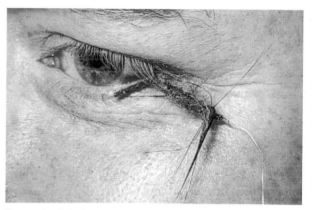

Penetrating injuries can be caused by fish hooks

Method of examination

- Check vision (count fingers, read signposts)
- Fields of vision to confrontation
- Examine the eye using a good light in a systematic fashion:
  Periorbital region
  External eye—conjunctiva; cornea; sclera (fluorescein drops)
  Intraocular contents—anterior chamber; pupil size, shape and reaction; posterior segment
  Eye movements

Indicators of serious injury

- Reduced vision
- Substantial pain
- Hyphaema
- Abnormality of pupil shape or function
- Marked subconjunctival haemorrhage or swelling
- Chemical material has entered the eye
- Diplopia

Arrange immediate referral to hospital if any doubt exists about the severity or nature of the injury

---

a drop of fluorescein that will stain a corneal foreign body or abrasion bright green. Corneal abrasions are extremely painful, and the player is unlikely to resume their game if one is sustained. Similarly, corneal foreign bodies will lead to suspension of play, as for these to be removed on the touchline is inappropriate. Topical antibiotic eye ointment should be instilled and a firm pad applied for those with a superficial eye injury. The upper eyelid should be everted with a cotton bud and any foreign material sitting under the lid swept off. More diffuse conjunctival material, such as mud, is best removed by irrigating the eye with sterile saline. Contact lens wearers should have the lens found and removed from the affected eye.

Hyphaema may be evident as a level of blood within the anterior chamber, but, more commonly in the acute phase, as a cloudy anterior chamber with a hazy appearance to the iris. The pupils should be equal, round, and reactive to light, and any irregularity should be considered a sign of intraocular damage.

Players with serious injuries should be transferred promptly to hospital for specialist attention. Before transfer, any chemical irritant should be washed out of the eye as a matter of urgency, and during transport the eye should be covered with a pad or plastic shield.

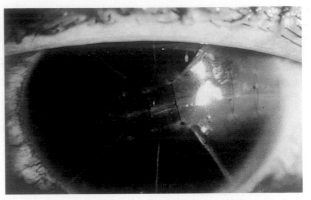

Repair of cornea after incisional refractive surgery. The eye had been struck by a squash racket causing rupture of the radial corneal refractive incisions that has been sutured

Methods of correcting vision

Twenty-five percent of all sportspeople need some form of refractive correction. The method chosen may affect the type and severity of injury sustained:

- Spectacles—simplest method and provide the best corrected vision and therefore should be used for high acuity sports(for example, shooting); may damage self or opponent in contact sports.
- Contact lenses—soft, large diameter lenses are relatively stable in the eye and are best for contact and combat sports.
- Hard lenses may shatter in the eye and not recommended.
- Refractive surgery—incisional surgery (radial keratotomy) is not performed now, but still may be people who have had it. Causes very weak eye and may have disastrous consequences.
- Surface based laser surgery (photorefractive keratectomy)— relatively safe and does not weaken the cornea.
- Intracorneal laser assisted in situ keratomileusis (flap and zap)—increasingly popular but is not compatible with contact sports for 6-12 months, as the superficial flap can become dislodged and lost.

Risk of injury is dependent on type of sport played

- Low risk—low velocity sports played on individual basis, without use of implements such as rackets, bats, sticks, or balls
- High risk—sports that use rapidly moving balls, sticks, and rackets or involve any degree of body contact. Such sports include the racket sports (squash, tennis, and badminton), football, rugby, cricket, and hockey
- Very high risk—combat sports, such as boxing and karate, by their very nature comprise a very high risk group for serious eye injuries

Sports associated with ocular trauma

A close relation exists between the type of sport and the risk of ocular injury. Frequency of injury depends, to some extent, on regional and national popularity: baseball is the most common cause of sports associated eye injury in the United States, hurling in Ireland, and football in the United Kingdom.

Protection and prevention

It is estimated that >90% of sports associated eye injuries are predictable and therefore avoidable. Prevention, therefore, is a priority. Strategies include:

- Education: teaching about the risks of injury and encouraging safe play by coaching and training.
- Regulation: ensuring that the rules of play are in the interest of eye safety.
- Protection: wearing protective eyewear for high risk sports. A British standard for eye protectors for squash is available. Well fitting eye protectors, made of clear, light polycarbonate material that is fog and scratch proof, have encouraged many

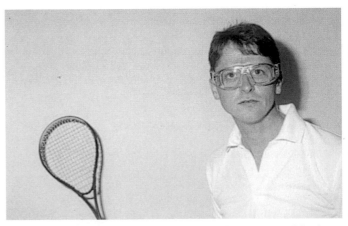

Eye protectors should be made of one piece of polycarbonate and fixed firmly to the head

players to wear them, and may have a prescription incorporated into the lenses to ensure good visual acuity.

- Prevention for high risk groups: screening to prevent those with high risk ocular conditions (for example, high myopia) or those who would be rendered visually handicapped if injured (for example, players with only one useful eye) from participating in the very high risk combat sports.

Summary

Eye injuries caused by sporting activities often are serious. The most frequent sports in the United Kingdom to cause serious eye injury are football, racket sports, rugby, and hockey.

When an injury is assessed, the doctor always should be aware of the circumstances and type of injury (for example, blunt or sharp), as this influences the type and extent of injury sustained. The eye should be examined systematically—bearing in mind that the lids should not be forced open.

Players need to see clearly to perform well—consider the method of visual correction used in the 25% of patients who have a refractive error, as this may affect the injury sustained. Refer immediately for a specialist opinion if a serious eye injury is suspected or if the player proves difficult to examine.

Prevention is better than cure. Always promote safe play and encourage the use of appropriate protective eye wear.

Further reading

- Vinger PF. Sports eye injuries: a preventible disease. *Ophthalmol* 1981;88:108-12
- MacEwen CJ. Sport-associated eye injuries: a casualty department survey. *Br J Ophthalmol* 1986;71:701-5
- Loran DFC, MacEwen CJ, eds *A textbook of sports vision*. Oxford: Butterworth Heinemann, 1995
- Zagelbaum BM, ed. *Sports ophthalmology*. Oxford: Blackwell Science, 1996
- Barr A, MacEwen CJ, Desai P, Baines PS. Ocular sports injuries: the current picture. *Br J Sports Exercise Med* 2000;34:456-8

The figure of cornea repair is reproduced with thanks to Dr G Crawford, Perth, Western Australia.

6 Groin pain

O J A Gilmore

Of all sports injuries, 5% are groin related. Accurate diagnosis often is difficult, because many pathological processes in and around the groin area can precipitate similar types of pain. The pain may be focal or diffuse. If not treated, the condition may become chronic and affect the patient's sports career. Although many activities can cause groin injuries, most are encountered in football, rugby, athletics, hockey, skating, cricket, running, equestrian, triathlon and general fitness training.

Aetiological factors

Hernia

Athletes who complain of pain in the groin rarely have a true hernia. An indirect inguinal hernia that becomes irreducible can produce groin pain. Patients with a direct inguinal hernia notice discomfort, particularly with prolonged standing or slow walking as opposed to more energetic sporting activities. Occasionally, a patient will have a femoral hernia and, rarely, an obturator hernia. Patients with an inguinal hernia have a palpable lump, with a cough impulse on standing, whereas femoral hernias are irreducible, presenting as a lump below and lateral to the pubic tubercle. Patients with symptomatic hernia need surgical repair.

Musculotendinous injuries

Soft tissue injuries account for most groin symptoms in sports people. Tendon injuries are often "overuse" injuries. Tendonitis is the result of an injury or degeneration of the tendon that results in an inflammatory reaction in the surrounding para-tendon. Rupture of the tendon, which can be partial or complete, may occur.

Adductor muscle strain

This is a common occurrence and is often a result of external rotation and abduction injuries, especially when the athlete does not warm up fully. High kicks and sliding tackles in football, repetitive abduction in ice skating, and horse riding predispose to adductor longus injuries. Onset of pain may follow a single incident or be insidious in origin. Pain in the groin is located in the adductor insertion region and exacerbated by ide separation of the legs. Tenderness around the origin of adductor longus in the pubic bone is characteristic. Symptoms are reproduced by resisted adduction.

Rectus abdominis strain

Sports events that involve repetitive flexion at the groin, such as sit ups and leg raises, may lead to rectus abdominis strain. Pain and tenderness is noted over the insertion of the muscle into the pubic bone. Symptoms are exacerbated by hip flexion against resistance or sit ups.

Iliopsoas strain

This can occur when the hip is actively flexed or when the hip is forcefully flexed against resistance. Repeated sit ups and rowing machine exercises are known to cause iliopsoas strain. Hip flexion against resistance may reproduce the symptoms.

Rectus femoris strain

The rectus femoris can be damaged at its origin on the upper half of the anterior inferior iliac spine. These injuries are often seen in association with sprint starts in runners and kicking

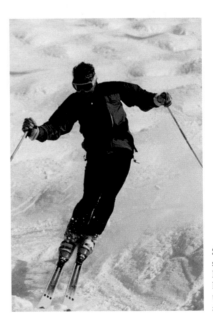

Skiing only causes adductor strains if the skier falls. People who ski properly keep their legs together and, therefore, tend not to get abduction injuries

episodes in football players. Pain and tenderness is noted over the muscle origin and exacerbated by resisted hip flexion.

Bursitis

Eight bursae are found around the hip joint in relation to attachment of the deep tendons. They can undergo inflammatory changes and can produce chronic groin pain. Bursitis is difficult to diagnose and is usually associated with muscular damage.

Inguinal ligament

Enthesopathy or inflammation at the insertion of the inguinal ligament in the pubic bone can also lead to chronic groin pain. Usually, the pain is diffuse and ill localised. This condition rarely exists alone.

Osteitis pubis

This condition, which is relatively uncommon, is related to instability and inflammation of the pubic symphysis. It is seen in adolescents and young adults who undertake vigorous exercise. Pain and tenderness is experienced over the pubic symphysis or along the pubic ramus.

Groin disruption (Gilmore's groin)

Groin disruption is a musculotendinous injury of the groin area that leads to chronic pain in athletes. Most patients are male soccer or rugby players, although other athletes may develop this problem. The pain in the inguinal region may inhibit or prevent the relevant sporting activity. It is also known as "Gilmore's groin" or "sports hernia".

Groin disruption occurs as an acute injury in one-third of patients, but it usually is an "overuse" injury. Repeated stretching of the posterior wall in the inguinal canal over long periods of time produces widening of the external ring because of tearing of the external oblique aponeurosis.

The conjoined tendon is formed by the union of the internal oblique and transversus abdominis muscle as a tendinous insertion at the pubic crease extending along the pectineal line. A torn conjoined tendon can be considered to be the same as a posterior wall defect at the medial margin of the inguinal canal region. Although musculotendinous disruption occurs, a proper hernial sac is not described as part of Gilmore's groin.

Degenerative changes of hip and spine

In some cases, osteoarthritis that affects the lumbosacral spine and hip joint can be responsible for chronic pain in the groin area. Intervertebral disc prolapse, which irritates the spinal nerve roots, can also lead to intractable groin pain.

Nerve entrapment

The ilioinguinal, iliohypogastric, genitofemoral, obturator, and lateral cutaneous nerve of the thigh can become involved in entrapment syndromes and may cause groin pain. Such incisions may be associated with nerve injury and subsequent entrapment or formation of neuromas. A local anaesthetic injection that relieves the pain may be used as a diagnostic test. In some patients, exploration of the area with excision of the involved nerve may be needed.

In other patients, high entrapment of the lateral cutaneous nerve of thigh in the fascia lata is a possible cause of groin pain, which can be relieved by surgical release. Gymnasts, in particular, can develop meralgia paraesthetica when practising on asymmetric bars because of entrapment of, or trauma to, the lateral cutaneous nerve of the thigh. A period of four to six weeks of an altered training programme usually allows the condition to settle.

> Trochanteric bursae and the bursae around the insertion of iliopsoas are most often involved in bursitis

---

Pathologies in groin disruption

- Torn external oblique aponeurosis, which produces a dilated superficial inguinal ring
- Torn conjoined tendon
- Dehiscence between conjoined tendon and inguinal ligament
- Absence of hernia sac

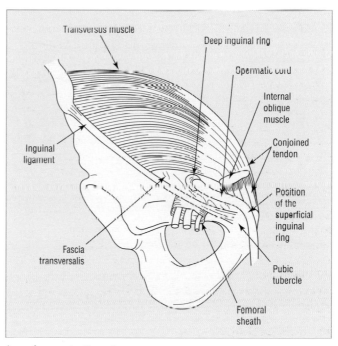

Area where groin disruption occurs

Groin disruption in professional football players

In studies on professional soccer players, the underlying problem in groin disruption is muscle imbalance and overuse. The strong hip flexors that are used to kick the ball tilt the pelvis forward; the forward pelvis stretches the abdominal muscles, which become weak and fail to stabilise the pelvis.

Excessive physical activity, especially twisting and turning, results in tears of the groin muscles, tendons, and ligaments and thus groin disruption. The underlying muscle imbalance means these patients may also have hamstring problems (recurrent tears) and back problems (often lordosis).

With appropriate training and core stability exercises, this balance can be corrected. The incidence of groin disruption over the past six years for one English premier football club's squad has substantially reduced since they started core stability exercises twice a week.

> Patients with nerve entrapment often have a history of previous surgery, such as appendicectomy, hernia repair, or a Pfannenstiel incision

Fractures

Rigorous sporting activities can lead to stress and avulsion fractures. Fractures that involve the pelvis and neck of the femur can lead to chronic or acute groin pain. Stress fractures increasingly are seen in long distance runners and joggers, especially women, and they usually affect the inferior pubic ramus close to the symphysis. Pain may be experienced in the groin, buttock, or thigh during or after training. Movements of the hip, particularly external rotation and abduction, are limited because of pain.

Plain radiographs may be negative in the initial weeks after a fracture. Pain is experienced in the groin and extends to the anterior thigh and sometimes to the knee. Compression fractures of the femoral neck are not uncommon. These are usually located at the medial margin of the cortex of the femoral neck and often are seen in younger athletes.

Slipped upper femoral epiphysis

This should be considered in adolescents as an uncommon cause of groin pain.

Investigations

Plain films

Plain films of the pelvis, hip joints, and lumbosacral spine will confirm the presence of fracture, avulsion, ectopic calcification, or degenerative change. In osteitis pubis, widening and fragmentation or sclerotic changes of the pubic symphysis are seen. Stork or flamingo views taken with the patient standing on one leg and then the other can show pelvic instability. If displacement is >3 mm, this may be important, and orthopaedic advice should be sought.

Ultrasound scanning

Ultrasound scanning may detect haematoma, cysts, hernia, varicocoele, hydrocoele, testicular, and intrapelvic pathology.

Bone scanning

Radioisotope bone scanning with technetium 99 can identify osteitis pubis, avulsion, and stress fractures, as well as early degenerative changes that affect the spine and other joints that may not show on plain radiograph.

Herniography

In this invasive investigation, contrast is introduced into the peritoneal cavity through a subumbilical puncture wound. The patient is then screened radiologically for evidence of a hernia sac. The procedure is useful in obscure or undetected hernias, but the success rate depends on the expertise of the radiologist. Herniography, however, is not diagnostic in groin disruption.

Magnetic resonance imaging

Magnetic resonance imaging of the pelvis and soft tissues of the groin are assuming an increasingly important role in the evaluation of the groin injuries. Magnetic resonance imaging can identify muscle and tendon injuries and bone and joint diseases and can give clues to groin disruption. Certain aspects of groin disruption, such as widening of the external ring in the inguinal canal and disruption of the external oblique, can be identified by an experienced radiologist, but magnetic resonance imaging remains more reliable for diagnosing injuries to the thigh than those in the inguinal region.

Appropriate investigations to exclude systemic pathology have to be considered. These include intravenous urography, cystoscopy, colonoscopy, computed tomography scanning and magnetic resonance imaging of the relevant areas.

> **Stress fractures of the femoral neck commonly are encountered in long distance runners, hurdlers, skiers, and football players**

Systemic causes of groin pain

Lower gastrointestinal disease
Diverticular disease, inflammatory bowel disease, appendicitis, mesenteric lymphadenitis and occasionally, bowel malignancies can give rise to groin pain but more usually pain in the iliac fossa.

Urological causes
Ureteric calculi, urinary tract infections, and prostatitis should be considered in the differential diagnosis.

Gynaecological causes
Chronic groin pain in women may be caused by pelvic inflammatory disease, endometriosis, or disease of the uterus, tubes of ovaries. Ultrasound scanning of the pelvis and referral to a gynaecologist is appropriate.

Testicular causes
Epididymo-orchitis, varicocoeles, trauma and occasionally, tumours can all cause groin pain. The history and examination will confirm a testicular cause. Ultrasound screening of the testes is useful for detecting small tumours, the most common form of malignancy in young men.

Inguinal lymphadenopathy
Tender inflamed inguinal lymph nodes, often secondary to abrasions on the leg, especially in soccer and rugby players may be the cause of groin pain.

Investigations

- Plain radiograph
  Hip and pelvis
  Stork (flamingo) views
- Bone scan (technetium 99)
- Ultrasound scan
  Groin and testes
  Pelvis
- Herniography
- Magnetic resonance image scan

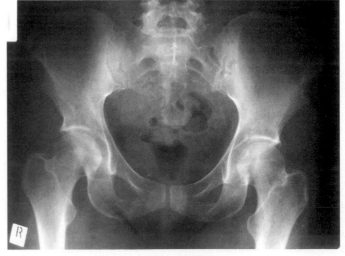

Radiograph of normal hip and pelvis of adult

Treatment

Musculotendinous injuries

"Groin strain" implies injury to any of the following muscles: the sartorius, any or all of the adductors (rider's strain), the long head of rectus femoris, the iliopsoas, and any of the abdominal muscles. A tear of the adductor muscles occurs around the musculotendinous junction about 5 cm from the pubis or at the tendo-osseus junction and produces pain around the pubic tubercle or superior ramus. Diagnosis is made by the presence of local tenderness, with pain on resisted contraction of isolated muscles. Chronic injuries are more difficult to evaluate and may involve more than one pathological process.

During the acute phase, the standard principles of soft tissue injury management should be followed for the first 48-72 hours. These include "functional" rather than complete rest if possible. Any activity that stresses the injured area should be avoided and crutches can be used in severe cases to limit use of the injured part. If possible, compression should also be applied and the injured area elevated. Analgesics or anti-inflammatory drugs are effective during the first 72 hours after injury.

Gentle movements within the limits of pain can begin following the acute phase, facilitating repair of the soft tissue. This phase of healing may last between 72 hours to six weeks. Passive and active stretching should be encouraged to limit muscle tightness. The patient's rehabilitation should begin as soon as pain allows.

At this stage, physiotherapeutic modalities may include massage, ultrasound, and electrical muscle stimulation, with clear instructions to the patient regarding limitation of the activity. When the repair phase is complete, the intensity of exercise is increased to permit tissue remodelling and a return to general fitness.

Surgery is indicated for the reattachment of serious avulsion injuries or repair of ruptured tendons or muscle tears.

Osteitis pubis is best managed by rest, the symptoms settling in several weeks or months. If there is substantial pelvic instability on weight bearing (>4 mm shift), plating or bone grafting may be considered.

Skeletal injuries

These require treatment by orthopaedic surgeons. Fractures can be treated conservatively if there is no serious distraction between bone ends. Sometimes internal fixation will be required followed by a rehabilitation programme.

Groin disruption

Conservative treatment, rest, and rehabilitation often fails, but surgical repair gives very good results. Surgery is indicated in professionals who cannot play or whose game is inhibited. In amateurs, surgery is indicated if everyday life is affected or if loss of sport affects the patient's quality of life. Exploration of the groin is performed through an inguinal incision, and each element of the disruption is identified and rectified. The conjoined tendon is repaired (2/0 polyglactic acid suture) and the transversalis fascia is repaired and plicated (2/0 polyglactic acid suture). If the rectus abdominis is torn, this is repaired with nylon (0 nylon). The key element of the repair is anchoring of the repaired conjoined tendon to the pubic tubercle with nylon and a tension free approximation of the repaired conjoined tendon to the inguinal ligament. The external oblique is then repaired (2/0 polyglactic acid suture) and the superficial inguinal ring reconstituted before the skin is closed with subcuticular dissolvable sutures. All professional athletes are given a rehabilitation programme of four weeks. Semi-professional and amateur athletes usually need an extra 1-2 weeks before returning to sport.

> Musculotendinous injuries can present acutely as a result of overstretching, twisting, or lunging

> Cooling of the injury with ice reduces hypoxic tissue damage and provides local analgesia. Ice packs should be applied 15-20 minutes every two hours for the first two days

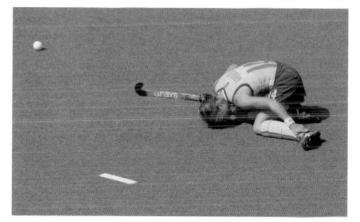

A musculotendinous injury in a hockey player. With permission from Getty Images

> Symptomatic inguinal or femoral hernias should be surgically repaired. Ice, mesh, or laparoscopic repair may be chosen according to individual preference. The aim is to achieve a tension free repair

---

Groin disruption rehabilitation programme

- Week 1— first day after operation: essential to stand upright and walk for 20 minutes. Then, walk gently four times a day. Follow gentle stretching exercises given by physiotherapists
- Week 2—jogging and gentle running in straight lines, gentle sit ups with knees bent. Adductor exercises—stretching and strengthening, step ups, cycling
- Week 3—increase speed to sprinting, increase sit ups and adductor exercises. Swimming (crawl)
- Week 4—sprint, twist and turn, kick, play

Summary

Groin pain is a considerable problem, especially in sportsmen rather than sportswomen. It often causes inability to participate and sometimes leads to retirement from sport. Professional sports players and manual workers may incur a loss of earnings because of restriction of activities. The psychological impact of being unable to play may lead to depression, especially if a financial loss is involved. The incidence of injury is increasing in elite sportsmen, who now take reduced breaks between seasons because of tours and other commitments. Doctors and physiotherapists increasingly are becoming aware of the significance and nature of groin injuries and the need to identify patients with groin disruption who will respond well to surgical repair, whereas in other athletes, it can be prevented by appropriate training and core stability exercises. Reports from different centres around the world indicate that with careful evaluation, appropriate rehabilitation, and surgical treatment when indicated, most sports players with groin injuries can be treated successfully and return to their previous level of sporting activity.

The radiograph of a normal hip is reproduced from *ABC of Emergency Radiology*, 2nd ed, with permission from WR Young and James AS Young.

Since 1980, 5344 sportsmen and 174 sportswomen have been referred to the author's injury clinic. Of these, 3246 men have needed surgery but only 33 women. That a return to elite sport is possible is shown by the successful treatment of 230 internationals football players from many countries, 52 rugby internationals (including three from England's world cup winning team), 18 cricketers, 13 hockey players, and a number of Olympic athletes

Further reading

- Gilmore OJA. Gilmores's groin. Ten years' experience of groin disruption—a previously unsolved sports problem. *Sports Med Soft Tissue Trauma* 1991;3:12-14
- Gilmore OJA. Groin pain in the soccer athlete: Fact, fiction and treatment. *Clin Sports Med* 1998;17:787-93
- Gilmore OJA. Groin disruption in sportsment. In: Kurzer M, Kark A, Wantz G, eds. *Surgical management of abdominal wall hernias*. London: Martin Dunitz, 1999:151-7
- Renstrom P. Tendon and muscle injuries in the groin area. *Clin Sports Med* 1992;11:815-31
- Urquhart DS, Packer GT, McLatchie GR. Return to sport and patient satisfaction levels after surgical treatment for groin disruption. *Sports Exer Inj* 1996;2:42

7 Management of injuries in children

> "Children, by their very nature, are biddable and as such are prey to the over ambitious parent and the over zealous coach"
>
> **JGP Williams**

JGP Williams's statement, of course, is not a statement that is universally appropriate, but the risk of that happening is real. It is extremely important to recognise that not all injuries lead to long term problems, but some do.

It is almost a cliché to say that children are not just little adults, but they are very different beings, and it is important in the understanding of their injuries to appreciate that they differ because they are growing. They are growing not only in their overall shape and size but also at a cellular level in the development of their bony skeleton. It is the effect of trauma on the developing skeleton that sets children's injuries apart. Growing bone is vulnerable to both acute and probably more importantly to overuse injuries. It is helpful in diagnosing children's injuries to "think bone" as the skeleton so often is involved in injuries. Some injuries can lead to asymmetrical growth and long term disabilities.

Most children, of course, take part in sport during their developing years without any serious problems as a result of their sporting activities. It is important, however, to recognise which injuries at least potentially can lead to disability.

Skeletal development

Skeletal development involves linear bone growth and skeletal maturation, as defined by bone age. Knowledge of these two processes is important in the understanding of skeletal injuries.

Linear growth

Linear growth decays exponentially with age, with the most rapid rate of growth being in the first year and the rate slowly reducing until skeletal maturation is reached. This fall is interrupted by the so-called mid growth spurt (not accepted by all observers) and the more important adolescent growth spurt.

The adolescent growth spurt is a time of risk of acute and overuse injury. The overall body shape is changing, and from being a compact well balanced individual, children tend to become rather gangly, less balanced, and rather uncoordinated. The child can take some time to adapt to this new shape, and it is a time when the risk of injury is high. The growth areas of the skeleton are active, somewhat weaker, and particularly vulnerable to injuries.

Skeletal maturation

Skeletal maturation depends on the rate of ossification of the cartilage scaffold and the pattern of appearance and then fusion of the ossification centres. Skeletal maturation is measured as bone age, by comparing a wrist radiograph with an atlas of wrist radiographs taken at different ages. The balance between linear growth and skeletal maturation determines a person's final adult stature.

Cartilage is converted into bone by endochondral ossification. This is an orderly process of cartilage cell division followed by the production of a matrix which then calcifies and is converted then into bone. The process can fail under stress,

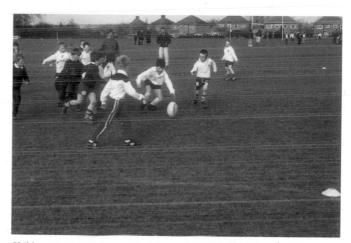

Children are put under great pressure when involved in sport at all levels

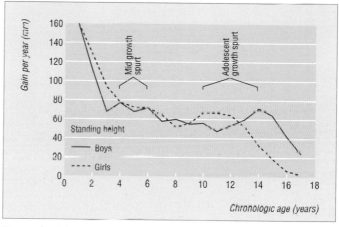

Linear growth in children

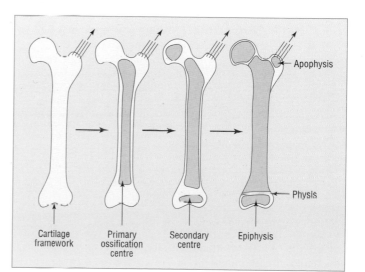

Endochondral ossification—shows conversion of cartilaginous scaffold into bone

leading to a group of conditions called osteochondroses. It takes place in the physes (growth plates), epiphyses (articular surfaces), and apophyses (tendon bone junctions).

Acute skeletal injuries

Tendon bone junctions

Children's tendons and ligaments can withstand trauma better than adults because they are more elastic and better vascularised and so are less likely to be affected by degenerate changes. It is more common to see avulsion fractures of the bone at a tendon or ligament insertion than to see soft tissue rupture.

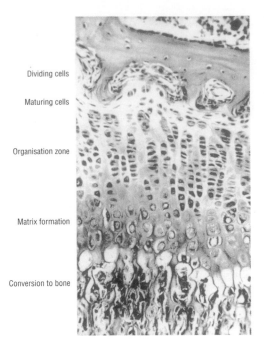

Dividing cells

Maturing cells

Organisation zone

Matrix formation

Conversion to bone

Endochondral ossification

Management of tendon bone junction injury

- The management can be active or conservative depending on the site and displacement of the fragment and also the age of the child
- Many avulsion fractures of the tibial spines for example can be managed by manipulation into extension and then immobilisation, but others may require internal fixation
- The outcome of these injuries should be good and even what might be seen as a significant displacement can indeed be accepted and healing can proceed without long term effects

---

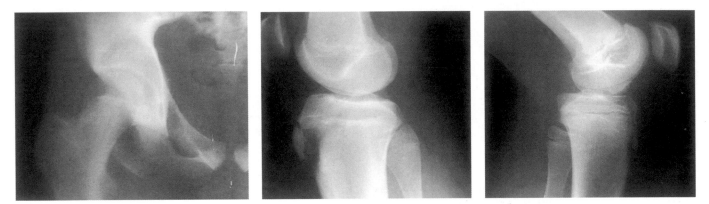

Acute bony avulsions: ischium (left), tibial tuberosity (middle), and tibial spine (right)

Shaft fractures

Fractures of the shaft of long bones usually are not worrying injuries, as long term consequences are rare.

Angulated fractures

These fractures are very forgiving and heal readily, with an ability to remodel, even if some degree of angulation exists. Remodelling is a long process. In young athletes, it may well be appropriate to reduce and immobilise the fracture if the angular deformity is great or if the fragments are displaced. Fixation with intramedullary nails or plates may then be needed.

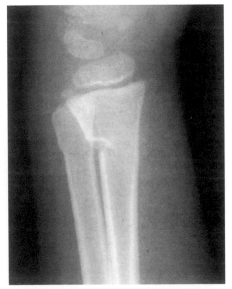

Buckle fracture

Management of angulated fractures

- Assessment of the angulation
- Manipulation and immobilisation with plaster of Paris
- Open reduction and internal fixation as appropriate
- Early mobilisation once the fracture has healed
- Physiotherapy to rehabilitate the limb

Buckle and greenstick fractures

These types of fracture usually are of no great concern as they heal readily. Immobilisation often is required only to achieve analgesia. They do require a period of rest, however, to allow fracture healing to take place.

Management of buckle and greenstick fractures

- Radiological assessment
- Appropriate immobilisation for pain relief
- Mobilisation once the fracture is pain free and has healed

Rotational deformities

Fractures that have a rotational element are very much more important. This deformity must be corrected or a permanent rotational deformity will result.

Supracondylar fractures of the humerus

These fractures are very important because of the potential for neurovascular damage. Careful assessment has to be made to identify this complication. When vascular damage has occurred, as evidenced by an absent peripheral pulse or signs of ischaemia, urgent operative intervention is needed.

Myositis ossificans is a frequent complication of this fracture. It involves the formation of calcium deposits in the capsule and soft tissues around the elbow joint, which eventually mature into bone. This leads to permanent loss of movement, which is of great importance in a sportsman who needs upper limb mobility. It is a difficult condition to prevent, but too early or aggressive rehabilitation can be a factor.

Fractured neck of femur

These are rare fractures. They have a high risk of avascular necrosis in the head, however, even a long time after the injury has occurred, resulting in permanent disability.

Articular fractures

These are significant injuries and can lead to long term problems such as long term osteoarthrosis. Anatomical reduction should be achieved, with internal fixation if necessary. Osteochondral fractures of an articular surface should be replaced and repaired if possible. Occasionally, the loose fragments need to be removed. These fractures can lead to non-participation in sport in the long term. The risk of developing degenerate changes in the affected joint is real.

Dislocations

Shoulder

This is a rare injury in children. A fracture of the physis of the upper humerus is more common than a dislocation. Shoulder dislocations carry a high risk of recurrent dislocation.

Patella

Patella dislocations and subluxations are common. Acute dislocations can be associated with an osteochondral lesion of the trochlea or patella, which may need surgical intervention. Recurrent dislocation is a complication and sometimes needs surgical intervention. It is common to find subluxing patellae and anterior patello-femoral knee pain.

Elbow

This common injury can sometimes be associated with fracture of the medial epicondyle after reduction of the dislocation. Myositis ossificans is not an uncommon complication.

Meniscal injuries

These are not common in children, but they do occur. An attempt should be made to retain as much of the torn meniscus as possible, and a meniscal suture should be attempted where at all possible. This will help prevent long term complications, such as osteoarthritis.

Physeal injuries

These are injuries to the physeal plate; if severe, they can permanently arrest growth in part or in all of the physis. These are common and have no equivalent in adults. The Salter-Harris classification of physeal fractures is a useful tool. Type I and type II fractures have an intact physeal plate, and

---

Management of rotational deformities

- Reduction of the fracture correcting the rotational deformity, followed by immobilisation with plaster or internal fixation
- Physiotherapy and rehabilitation after fracture union

Management of supracondylar fractures of the humerus

- Early recognition of neurovascular complications and surgical management
- Anatomical reduction with or without internal fixation to correct any rotational deformity
- Gentle mobilisation once fracture union is achieved
- Active but not passive exercises should be encouraged

Management of fractured neck of femur

- Internal fixation
- Restricted weight bearing until fracture union
- Careful monitoring and long term follow up to identify any complications

Management of articular fractures

- Early recognition
- Surgical intervention usually is necessary to reduce or fix the fracture or remove any loose bodies
- Immobilisation without weight bearing on the joint until fracture union
- Progressive rehabilitation

Management of dislocations

Shoulder
- The dislocation should be reduced and may be associated with a stabilisation procedure by operative intervention

Patella
- Acute dislocation should be reduced and the limb immobilised for three weeks
- Appropriate rehabilitation with physiotherapy in terms of muscle re-education

Elbow
- Radiograph assessment to identify associated fractures
- Closed manipulation reduction, with possible fixation of any fracture
- Rest in a splint while swelling settles followed by gentle mobilisation exercises
- Look for myositis ossificans
- Graduated activities
- Explanation that recovery may be a long term problem in terms of achieving mobility

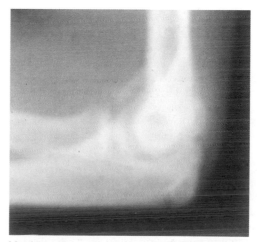

Myositis ossificans, showing calcification in the anterior capsule of the joint

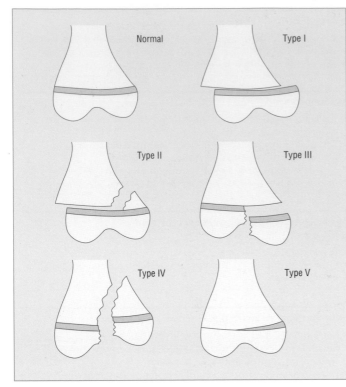

Salter-Harris classification of fractures

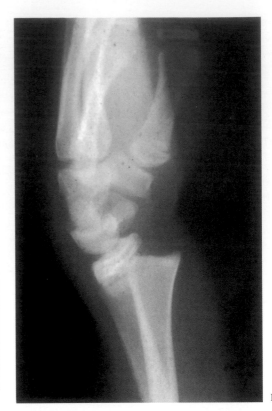

Physeal fracture

the prognosis is very good. Closed reduction of the fracture should ensure normal physeal growth. In type III and type IV fractures, the physeal plate is disrupted, and this must be reduced anatomically. Without anatomical reduction, union of the epiphysis to the metaphysis preventing the physis growing is a risk, and asymmetrical growth can follow. This can lead to deformity that may need correcting. Type V fractures are injuries to the physeal plate and, if severe, can permanently arrest growth in part or all of the physis. These can be difficult fractures to diagnose even with X-ray control.

Overuse skeletal injuries

These occur due to fatigue of the bone and not as a direct result of injury. The symptoms often can be ignored, leading to a much longer healing process. The view that there is "no gain without pain" should be challenged, particularly where children are involved, as long term damage can be done.

The best treatment is rest. It is very difficult, however, for coaches, parents, and young performers to accept this. It requires a very responsible attitude to be adopted. Overuse injuries in children are more likely to affect the skeleton than the soft tissues. It is important to "think bone," so that problems that affect skeletal growth are not overlooked. The pathological change that occurs is a denaturing of the process of endochondral ossification, such that fragmentation of the bone occurs, followed by revascularisation and healing. All these injuries will heal, but the position, state, and condition of the way in which they heal can lead to permanent disability.

Apophyseal injury (tendon bone junction injury)

Fractures at tendon bone junctions are often referred to by eponyms, such as Osgood-Schlatter's disease (pull of the patella tendon on the tibial tuberosity that can lead to its fragmentation). Other common sites are the lower pole of the patella (Sinding-Larsen-Johannson disease) and the os calcis apophysis (Sever's disease), where the Achilles' tendon is inserted.

Management of physeal injuries

- Early recognition and assessment of the injury
- Anatomical reduction of the physis is needed, particularly if the fracture crosses the plate, as this often needs surgical intervention
- Immobilisation
- Rehabilitation
- Careful monitoring to identify any abnormality of subsequent growth

---

Management of tendon bone junction injuries

- Recognition and early diagnosis—"think bone"
- Careful explanation of the condition
- Rest and restriction of activity involving the affected part—for example, rebound activities with Osgood Schlatter's disease. Complete restriction of activity sometimes is needed, and splintage to immobilise the part may be helpful
- Arrange training around the injury, with care not to produce an injury of a different area because of overconcentration of activity
- Physiotherapy to address muscle balance to gently stretch the affected muscle. Care is needed not to adversely affect the condition
- Reassurance that resolution is virtually certain but needs patience

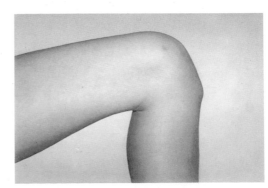

Osgood-Schlatter's disease

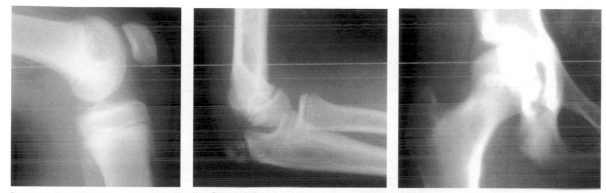

Common sites of apophyseal injuries: Sinding-Larsen-Johannson disease (left), olecranon apophysitis (middle), and ischial tuberosity (right)

Injuries to the base of the fifth metatarsal can result from a pull of the peroneus brevis inserted there; they occur in sports where balance particularly is required. The ischial tuberosity can be affected by the pull of hamstrings and the anterior superior iliac spine by the pull of the sartorius. Indeed, the whole iliac crest apophysis can be affected by the pull of the abdominal muscles. In sports that involve the upper limbs, such as gymnastics, the olecranon epiphysis can fracture.

Diagnosis of these conditions is often clinical, but radiograph confirmation is sometimes needed. Often radiological changes are seen. These conditions occur most commonly at the time of the growth spurt, when the apophyses are relatively weak and the muscles relatively tight, as they grow in length less quickly than the bone. Times of increased activity in training or competition can also be a factor.

Tendon bone junction injuries are recognised by point tenderness at the muscle insertion. They often are overlooked, however, because of their insidious onset and the fact that the pain initially does not interfere with the ability to perform. Early diagnosis is helpful in reducing the time taken for the condition to heal. The natural history is for complete recovery, the only question is the time it takes to achieve this.

Epiphyseal injuries (articular osteochondrosis)

The term osteochondritis dissecans is used to denote this group of fairly uncommon injuries. In the lower limb, the knee is the most common site, although such injuries can occur in the talus and occasionally the hip joint. In the upper limb, this type of injury occurs in the capitellum of the humerus and is seen in children who participate in sports such as gymnastics and those that involve compressive strains on the elbow joint. Sometimes, the whole capitellum can be affected and becomes avascular; this is termed "Panner's disease." This presents initially as an achy joint, which is slowly progressive, but in the early stages, it is often possible to work through the discomfort. In the lower limb, a limp often is present, whereas in the elbow joint, one of the early signs is loss of full extension to the joint. An effusion often is the first clinical sign to appear. Pain is progressive and eventually leads to locking if a loose body forms. Any child who presents with a painful joint must be investigated very carefully.

The compressive forces on the convex surface of the joint lead to an avascular segment that can separate from the underlying bone. The diagnosis is made by having a suspicion from the history and on clinical examination; this can be confirmed by imaging. Radiographs usually show the involved segment, and a magnetic resonance imaging scan is helpful, particularly in identifying whether the overlying articular cartilage is intact. If the diagnosis is made early, the condition may not necessarily progress; it can heal and leave a congruous joint such that normal activities can be resumed. The joint surface may become softened and deformed, however, because of collapse of the underlying bone and early arthrosis results.

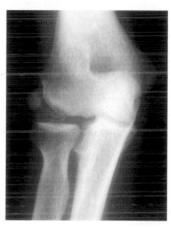

Epiphyseal injury in the capitellum of the humerus

> **Why articular osteochondrosis occurs in some children and not others is unclear, but a hereditary link may exist**

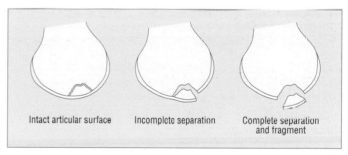

Intact articular surface   Incomplete separation   Complete separation and fragment

Osteochondritis dissecans—shows different stages that epiphyseal injuries can go through: from avascular segment with articular surface through segment with partial separation of fragment to complete separation of segment such that it forms a loose body

Management of articular osteochondrosis injury

- Early recognition—"think bone"
- In the early stages with an intact articular surface, a period of non-weight bearing is needed if the symptoms are severe
- Complete restraint from sporting activities of rebound and twisting
- Slow increase in activities can be allowed, as long as no symptoms recur. Careful follow up is essential, with imaging, as needed, to identify the progression of healing
- Arthroscopic assessment can often be needed if symptoms persist. With partial separation of the fragment, operative intervention to fix the fragment back in place can be needed. This should be followed by careful follow up as advised
- Once a loose body is diagnosed, surgical removal is necessary. Later consideration of chondral grafting techniques may be appropriate

The natural history of healing of articular osteochondrosis may take 18 months or more. In some sports, this may curtail a patient's ability to participate and achieve

Physeal injuries (growth plate osteochondrosis)
Upper limb
Physeal failure under stress is relatively rare. It occurs in the upper limb where the area of the physeal plates is smaller than those in the lower limb and so can be more vulnerable to stress in sports that involve weight bearing and rebound. A stress reaction can be seen in the olecranon physis, and the distal radial physis is also vulnerable in gymnasts. The child presents with pain in the area, accompanied by local tenderness and swelling around the physis. Radiographs show widening of the physeal plate, and gross changes often are seen in the wrist, with scalloping and failure of calcification. The prognosis is good if diagnosed early. Growth can be interrupted, however, and the radius may finish shorter than the ulna. This may need surgical treatment, but this complication is relatively rare.

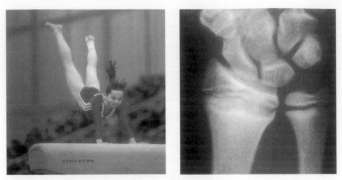

Rebound activity (left) and widening of the distal radial physis (right)

Management of upper limb physeal injuries (growth plate osteochondrosis injury)
- Diagnosis is clinical and radiological— "think bone"
- Strict curtailment of upper limb activities, maybe for three months
- Careful monitoring of healing process
- Gradual reintroduction of activity once healing is complete

Spinal
Osteochondrosis of the spine occurs as a result of flexion forces acting on the anterior part of the vertebral body. The anterior growth plate is damaged, and the vertebrae may become wedged, resulting in a kyphotic spinal deformity. This can occur in the thoracic and lumbar spines, and is more common in children with tight hamstrings.

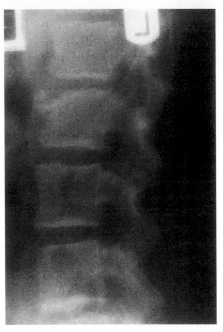

Spinal osteochondritis lumbar vertebrae

Management of spinal physeal injuries (growth plate osteochondrosis injury)
- Early radiological diagnosis
- Rest
- Careful review to identify any kyphotic deformity
- Slow, progressive activity once symptoms settle
- Gradual reintroduction of sporting activity

Stress fractures
Stress fractures of the long bones and other parts of the skeleton occur in children just as they do in adults and should be treated in the same way. A stress fracture of the pars intra-articularis of the lamina of the spinal vertebra, however, is common in children, especially adolescents. The injury is caused by extension and rotational stresses. The defect in the lamina is initially just a stress reaction and cannot be seen

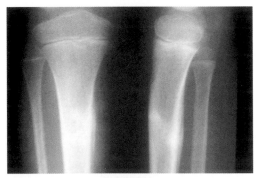

Stress fracture of the tibia in a child

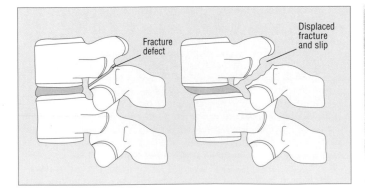

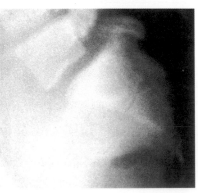

Stress fracture of the pars intra-articularis (left) and x ray showing vertebral slip (right)

radiologically; bone scanning techniques or reverse gantry computed tomography scanning is needed to pick up the injury at that stage. Alternatively, pars specific magnetic resonance imaging sequences may detect these lesions and reduce radiation exposure in children.

Stress reaction to the bone can develop to form a bony defect known as spondylolysis, which can be followed by a forward slip of the affected vertebra on the vertebra below—a condition known as a spondylolisthesis. Prognosis generally is good, and surgical intervention is not usually needed.

The cross-sectional illustration of endochondral ossification is taken from Ham AW, Lesson TS. *HAM histology*, Pitman Medical Publishing Co. Ltd, London (a JB Lippincott company), 1961. The Salter-Harris classification of fractures illustration is taken from *Injuries involving the epiphyseal plate* by Salter-Harris in *Journal of Bone and Joint Surgery* 1963;55a:587-622. The diagram of linear growth in children is taken from Dughie RB. *Clinical Orthopaedics* 1959;14:7-18. The endochondral ossification diagram was first published in *A Level 2 Course National Coaching Foundation Leads*.

Stress fractures occur in children across virtually the whole sporting spectrum, with high incidences reported in gymnastics, cricket, and rugby

Management of stress fracture

- Appropriate diagnosis
- Absolute rest from activities
- Appropriate stabilisation exercises
- Careful monitoring
- Gradual reintroduction of activities
- Injection techniques sometimes can be helpful
- Spinal fusion may be needed if the defect does not heal and remains symptomatic

8 Exercise induced asthma

Mark Harries, John Dickinson

The airways' normal physiological response to a period of exercise is dilatation. This bronchial dilatation shows as an increase in peak expiratory flow rate or forced expiratory volume in one second and is evident for up to an hour after exercise stops. This is thought to be an adaptive response to satisfy the demands for higher minute ventilation. By contrast, in about 80% of all people with asthma, the situation is reversed, with expiratory limitation associated with smooth muscle contraction, airway inflammation, and mucus production developing maximally about 10 minutes after exercise stops. Exercise induced asthma is characterised by a broad spectrum of symptoms, including wheezing, coughing, tight chest, dyspnoea, and excess mucus production. The association between a history of asthma and expiratory limitation induced by exercise is so strong that an exercise challenge may be used whenever the diagnosis of asthma is in doubt.

Need for spirometric evidence for exercise induced asthma

Since the 1984 Olympic games in Los Angeles, the number of athletes claiming to need inhaled drugs has seen an extraordinary rise. This varies between sports and is highest among swimmers and cyclists. An increased use of inhalers is among the reasons the International Olympic Committee made the following statement: "any athlete who wishes to use inhaled medication (steroid or bronchodilator) to treat an asthmatic condition in Olympic competition must produce evidence through results from either a bronchodilator or provocation test (such as exercise or histamine and methacholine challenge). For the test to be valid it must contain quantitative and graphic evidence, from a spirometer that is endorsed to American Thoracic Society standards." The athlete must also provide a letter from the attending physician stating the drugs being taken and in what dosage. This ruling was enforced at the 2004 Summer Olympic Games in Athens, and similar guidelines are being introduced by international governing bodies such as the International Association of Athletics Federations.

Diagnosis

Inhaled β agonist

For a person with normal airways, an inhaled short acting β_2 agonist shows no effect, but bronchial dilatation is the characteristic response of nearly all asthmatics. A rise in forced expiratory volume in one second of 15% or more 10 minutes after inhaling a short acting β_2 agonist is diagnostic, thus obviating the need for a provocation test.

Provocation tests

Exercise challenge

The International Olympic Committee regards an exercise test as positive if forced expiratory volume in one second decreases by ≥10% any time within 30 minutes of exercise stopping. Maximum effort flow loops should be measured before exercise and afterwards, at 3, 5, 10, 15, 20, and 30 minutes. Exercise challenges can be sport specific or involve an intense piece of exercise (>80% maximum heart rate) lasting ≥6 minutes. Exercise challenges conducted in the laboratory should be avoided, as a false negative test may occur.[1] If possible, the

Incidence of exercise induced asthma in elite sport

Incidence of exercise induced asthma can vary dramatically. Sports that take place in cold environments seem to have a higher incidence than other sports. The same is true for those who exercise in chlorinated pools.

Sport	Incidence (%)
Athletics	25
Hockey	33
Swimming	44
Cycling	44
Rowing	20
Great Britain Olympic Squad 2000	21*
Cross country skiing	50†
Figure skating	21†

*Data from Great Britain Olympic Squad for the Sydney Olympics 2000
†Data from Wilber et al. *Med Sci Sport Exercise* 2000;32:732-7

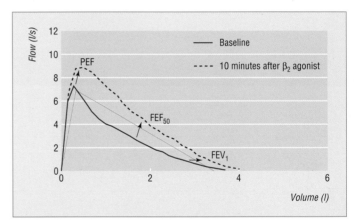

Positive bronchodilator challenge—expiratory flow rate in person with asthma 10 minutes after inhaling 200 µg of salbutamol (a short acting β_2 agonist). PEF (peak expiratory flow), FEF_{50} (forced expiratory flow at 50% of vital capacity) and FEV_1 (forced expiratory volume in one second) all rise. A rise of >15% FEV_1 meets the criteria set by international sporting governing bodies to justify the use of β_2 agonists in competition

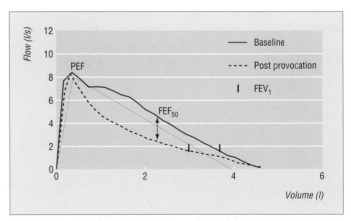

Exercise induced asthma positive provocation challenge—after the challenge PEF remains the same. FEV_1 and FEF_{50} fall and there is scalloping of the curve. The drop in FEF_{50} is greater than the drop in FEV_1

exercise challenge should best match the environmental conditions encountered by the athlete.

Eucapnic voluntary hyperpnoea challenge

Eucapnic voluntary hyperpnoea challenges are designed to simulate breathing rate and volume at about 85% of maximum voluntary ventilation (30 times forced expiratory volume in one second). The participant is asked to hyperventilate at 85% maximum voluntary ventilation for six minutes, which is only made possible by adding 5% carbon dioxide to the inhaled gas. Flow loop measurements should be taken at the same time periods for the exercise challenge. The International Olympic Committee defines a positive test as a fall in forced expiratory volume in one second of ≥10% within 30 minutes.

Eucapnic voluntary hyperpnoea challenges are regarded by some as the "gold standard."[2] The test is relatively expensive, however, and the apparatus must be built specially. At the Olympic Medical Institute, eucapnic voluntary hyperpnoea is used as a research tool and in elite athletes whose outdoor exercise challenge fails to elicit a substantial fall in forced expiratory volume in one second despite important symptoms.

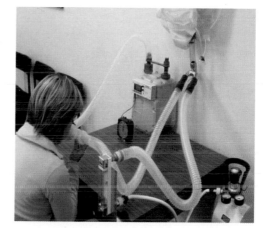

Athlete during a eucapnic voluntary hypernoea challenge. The athlete can see the clock, dry meter, and reservoir bag during the challenge. Verbal feedback during the test is given at least every minute, and ideally every 30 seconds. The feedback should include information about the current breathing rate and whether it should increase, decrease, or remain the same to achieve the target of 30 × FEV_1 for six minutes

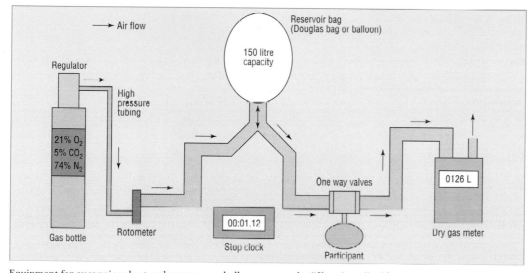

Equipment for eucapnic voluntary hyperpnoea challenge—note the 5% carbon dioxide concentration in gas to prevent the participant breathing off carbon dioxide during hyperventilation. The rate the gas passes to the participant is set through the rotometer (30 × FEV_1). The volume of the air breathed out by the participant is recorded at the dry gas meter. Actual breathing rate is calculated using the stop clock and dry gas meter taking readings every minute. If the breathing rate is not matched the remaining air will collect in the reservoir bag, causing the bag to increase in size. The air flow must be lowered at the rotometer if the bag fills much (target breathing rate does not alter)

Histamine and methacholine challenges

A feature common to all asthmatics, and some symptomless individuals, is an overall increase in the sensitivity of the bronchial tree to inhaled histamine or methacholine. This increased responsiveness is expressed as dose (mg/ml) that induces 20% decrease in forced expiratory volume in one second or peak expiratory flow rate; it is known as the histamine or methacholine PC20. The greater the reactivity, the smaller the dose needed to provoke a response. People with this so called bronchial hyper-reactivity also respond adversely to environmental pollutants, such as nitric oxide or ozone, in a way that those with normal airways do not. The International Olympic Committee's definition of a positive histamine and methacholine challenge varies depending on the length of time an athlete has taken corticosteroids. Thus, before a positive diagnosis is made, a thorough check of the International Olympic Committee's regulations must be made to ensure the athlete has met the criteria. Histamine and methacholine challenges are useful clinically to identify people who have hyper-reactive airways. As they are not specific to exercise, they should not be the first line for diagnosis.

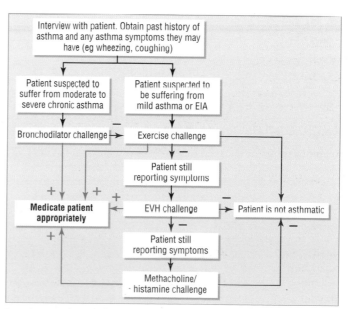

Exercise induced asthma diagnosis. (EIA = exercise induced asthma; EVH = eucapnic voluntary challenge)

Shape of maximum effort expiratory flow loop

Forced expiratory volume in one second and peak expiratory flow rate are used as measurements of airflow obstruction, whether reversible, as in asthma, or irreversible, as in chronic bronchitis. Both measurements depend on the volume of the initial breath taken and also on the effort put into expiration. It is possible for an unscrupulous person to fake exercise induced asthma by taking a smaller breath for the post-exercise measurement and so careful supervision of the test procedure is essential. However, a feature of all patients with obstructive airways disease, reversible or not, is the increased effort required to breathe out, with the result that smaller airways that are unsupported by cartilage collapse. This produces highly typical scalloping of the forced expiratory loop. As a result, the percentage fall in forced expiratory flow at 50% (FEF_{50}) is greater than the fall in either forced expiratory volume in one second or peak expiratory flow in one second. This scalloping cannot be faked and may provide a diagnostic clue when perusing the flow loops who are thought to have exercise induced asthma, but are relatively free of symptoms. It must be remembered that for diagnosis of exercise induced asthma the International Olympic Committee and other governing bodies do not recognise falls in FEF_{50} post provocation challenge.

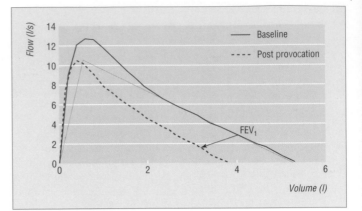

Negative exercise induced asthma flow loop—FVC, FEV_1, PEF, and FEF_{50} fall after exercise but the shape of the curve remains the same. The participant has taken a smaller breath after exercise

Measurement of forced expiratory volume with spirometer

- Stop all inhalers before test:
    Short acting β_2 agonists 12 hours before
    Long acting β_2 agonists 48 hours before
    Corticosteroids 72 hours before
- If patients experience any distressful asthma problems, they should restart their drugs. This will mean that they will be unable to complete any test for asthma
- Spirometer that meets American Thoracic Society Standards should be used
- Patient must be sitting down to avoid syncope during forced expiratory manoeuvres
- Nose clip must be worn to prevent air escaping through nose
- Patients must take at least three normal breaths before they are instructed to inspire fully
- Expiration should be as hard and fast as possible and to the fullest extent
- Ideally, three flow loops are needed for every measurement point. The flow loop with the best forced expiratory volume in one second should be recorded, as long as the variance between flow loops is not greater than 5%
- Only one test should be carried out each day, as maximal expiratory and inspiratory manoeuvres are fatiguing and false results could be drawn

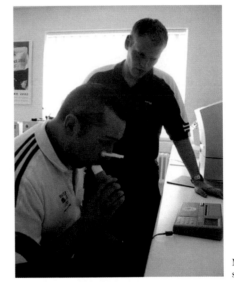

Measurement with a spirometer

Treatment

Regulations about drugs in tablet form remain in force, and all systemic oral medication is banned with the exception of aminophyllin. At the time of writing, all long acting β agonists are restricted, but the situation is fluid and likely to change.

Inhaled corticosteroids

Treatment with inhaled steroids forms the mainstay for all patients with asthma. Dry powder preparations are preferred to metered dose inhalers, largely because their use depends less on technique. Each uses a different delivery system, fluticasone uses an Accuhaler, budesonide a Turbohaler and mometasone a Twisthaler. A trend towards once daily treatment taken in the evening is being seen, although more symptomatic people may need treatment twice daily.

Further reading

- Rundell K, Wilber R, Lemanske R, eds. *Exercise-induced asthma: pathophysiology and treatment.* Illinois: Human Kinetics Publishers Inc, 2002
- Storms W. Review of exercise-induced asthma. *Med Sci Sports Exercise* 2003;35:1464-70
- Rundell K, Spiering B. Inspiratory stridor in elite athletes. *Chest* 2003;123:468-74
- Anderson S. Exercise-induced asthma in children: a marker of airway inflammation. *Med J Australia* 2002;177:S61-3
- Mickleborough T, Gotshall R. Dietary components with demonstrated effectiveness in decreasing the severity of exercise-induced asthma. *Sports Med* 2003;33:671-81
- Langdeau J, Boulet L. Prevalence and mechanisms of development of asthma and airway hyperresponsiveness in athletes. *Sports Med* 2001;31:601-16
- Joos G, Connor B. Indirect airway challenges. *Eur Resp J* 2003;21:1050-68
- Rundell K, Im J, Mayers L, Wilber R, Szmedra L, Schmitz H. Self-reported symptoms and exercise induced asthma in the elite athlete. *Med Sci Sports Exercise* 2001;33:208-13
- Helenius I, Haahtela T. Allergy and asthma in elite summer sport athletes. *J Allergy Clin Immunol* 2000;106:444-52

Inhaled β agonists

Inhaled β agonists supplement steroid treatment. Short acting preparations may need to be taken as often as four times daily, with an additional dose taken 10 minutes before competition. A typical declaration might be worded as follows: "Joe Bloggs is a patient of mine with exercise induced asthma for which he takes budesonide 400 µg at night and terbutaline 500 µg four times a day. Flow loops recorded before and 10 minutes after exercise are enclosed."

Sodium cromoglycate

Sodium cromoglycate inhibits exercise induced asthma when inhaled 10 minutes before exercise. It is especially effective in children, for whom it provides a useful alternative to steroids. No declaration is required.

1 Rundell KW, Wilber RL, Szmedra L, Jenkinson DM, Mayers LB, Im J. Exercise-induced asthma screening of elite athletes: field versus laboratory exercise challenge. *Med Sci Sports Exercise* 2000;32:309-16

2 Anderson SD. Provocation by eucapnic voluntary hyperpnoea to identify exercise induced bronchoconstriction. *Br J Sports Med* 2001;35:344-47

9 Infections

Geoffrey Pasvol

Several factors predispose sportspeople to infection, including: reduced immunity resulting from stress and overtraining, close contact with others, trauma (especially of the skin), foreign travel, and sexual activity, with its concomitant risks of diseases, such as hepatitis B and HIV.

Upper respiratory tract infections

Upper respiratory tract infections are of concern to athletes, especially when they are recurrent. They are commonly due to viruses, such as enteroviruses (echovirus and coxsackie), adenoviruses, and influenza virus, and β haemolytic streptococci. *Chlamydia pneumoniae*, which can lead to myocarditis, has gained notoriety in Swedish orienteers. Rapid methods are available to distinguish these conditions from one another, such as throat culture for β haemolytic streptococci or heterophile antibody (Paul-Bunnell) test for infectious mononucleosis. Viral culture and serology in diagnosis seldom are helpful, although such tests might confirm past infection.

Symptomatic relief with analgesics, antihistamines, or decongestants may help in some cases, although care is advised in selection of drug to avoid a doping infringement. Group A β haemolytic streptococcal sore throat is treated with penicillin, or a second generation cefalosporin or erythromycin in patients with penicillin allergy. Treatment should continue for at least 10 days to avoid recurrence.

Routes of spread

Whether or not a person with an upper respiratory tract infection should refrain from exercise is a major issue. In the presence of fever, tachycardia at rest, or severe myalgia or lethargy, athletes should not participate in sport. Complications such as cardiac arrhythmias have been overemphasised. Viral myocarditis is a rare event. Sudden cardiac death is more often the result of hypertrophic cardiomyopathy or undetected coronary artery disease.

The glandular fevers include infectious mononucleosis (caused by Epstein-Barr virus), toxoplasmosis, cytomegalovirus infection and, more recently, HIV seroconversion illness. *ITCH*

Infectious mononucleosis

Infectious mononucleosis caused by Epstein-Barr virus is an important and common infection in athletes. Spread is mainly via intimate close contact; thus isolation of proven or suspected cases is unnecessary.

Laboratory diagnosis of infectious mononucleosis is made on the basis of a significant number of atypical lymphocytes (>15%) on the peripheral blood film. A heterophile antibody test for the condition, such as the Monospot test, may be negative in the first week or two of illness and remains negative throughout in about 15% of cases.

The serum may also be tested for antibodies against the viral capsid antigen. A positive test for viral capsid antigen immunoglobulin M confirms current or recent infection. A positive test for viral capsid antigen immunoglobulin G (whatever the titre) in the absence of a positive immunoglobulin M indicates only past infection.

Infectious mononucleosis lasts for about 2-6 weeks and generally is self-limiting. The use of corticosteroids in infectious

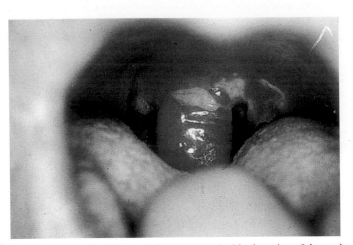

Pharyngitis caused by β haemolytic streptococci, with ulceration of the uvula

---

Common clinical presentations of infection with Epstein-Barr virus

- Sore throat with fever and generalised lymphadenopathy, with or without enlarged spleen
- In a few cases, diffuse maculopapular rash may be present
- Patients may present with hepatic illness with jaundice
- Haematological disorder (such as thrombocytopenia, haemolytic anaemia, or pancytopenia)
- Any neurological disorder ranging from encephalitis to peripheral neuropathy

---

Complications of infection with Epstein-Barr virus of particular relevance to athletes

- Splenic rupture—up to 40% of cases of traumatic splenic rupture have occurred in athletes who have, or have subsequently been found to have, infectious mononucleosis
- Persistent fatigue—in a few cases, fatigue and lethargy may persist for an indefinite period. These cases may include a proportion of people with chronic fatigue syndrome
- Myocarditis with persistent tachycardia, abnormal electrocardiogram, and raised cardiac enzymes

---

Routes of spread of infection

Young sportspeople are most susceptible to infections spread by:
- Droplets—for example, upper respiratory tract infections
- Orofaecal route—for example, traveller's diarrhoea and hepatitis A and E
- Water—for example, Leptospirosis
- Direct contact—for example, herpes simplex virus and impetigo
- Wound infection—for example, tetanus and streptococcal or staphylococcal infections
- Sexual activity—for example, hepatitis B and HIV
- Insect vectors—for example, malaria, Lyme disease

mononucleosis has been established only in the case of obstructive pharyngitis, whereas the usefulness of corticosteroids in cases with liver, neurological, or haematological involvement is unproven. Corticosteroids have not been shown to reduce the risk of splenic rupture or fatigue. Return to sporting activity after infectious mononucleosis should always be graded and limited to the exercise tolerance of the patient. Total bed rest is unnecessary and may even delay recovery. As the risk of splenic rupture is greatest in the first months after infection, strenuous exercise and alcohol consumption should be avoided during this period, especially in those who participate in contact sports.

Toxoplasmosis

Toxoplasma gondii, an intracellular protozoan infection acquired from cats and undercooked or raw meat, may produce a glandular fever syndrome with fever, hepatosplenomegaly, and generalised or localised lymphadenopathy. The clinical diagnosis of toxoplasmosis can be confirmed by serology and a fourfold rise or fall in the toxoplasma latex test, or a positive toxoplasma IgM, regardless of titre, is indicative of recent infection. Most episodes of toxoplasmosis are self-limiting and people who are not immunocompromised do not need to receive specific treatment.

Cytomegalovirus

Glandular fever syndrome, with or without jaundice, caused by cytomegalovirus is uncommon and usually self-limiting.

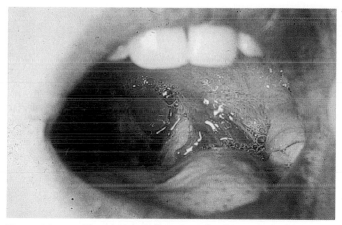

Pharyngitis caused by the Epstein-Barr virus, showing a pale membrane

Hepatitis

Hepatitis A

Nausea, loss of appetite, vomiting, and abdominal pain in hepatitis A often precede the appearance of jaundice by a number of days and the person is most infectious during this period. The urine becomes dark because of the presence of bilirubin and the stools light because of intrahepatic cholestasis. Jaundice may then appear and remain for a few days or weeks, followed by a variable period until complete recovery. Hepatitis A is contagious and spreads rapidly. Close contacts should be given passive protection with 250 mg intramuscular γ globulin. By the time jaundice appears, however, the need to isolate the patient has passed. Diagnosis is confirmed in the laboratory with a hepatitis A virus immunoglobulin M antibody test. The illness can be monitored by the measurement of liver function, such as through the transaminases and lactate dehydrogenase, but these do not necessarily correlate with the severity of disease or outcome. Hepatitis A virus immunoglobulin G indicates past infection only. The major risk in hepatitis A is that of fulminant acute liver failure, which occurs in <1% of cases. Some patients may have minor but generally short lived relapses.

Hepatitis B

Prodromal symptoms of hepatitis B are similar to those of hepatitis A, but they may occasionally be preceded by a skin rash or arthralgia, or both. Treatment of acute cases is symptomatic and more than 90% recover spontaneously. Careful follow up of patients with hepatitis B virus infection is important to ensure they do not develop any important sequelae. At present, no evidence shows that chronic carriers of hepatitis B virus should not participate in sport, except in close contact sports such as boxing, wrestling, and rugby, when skin wounds or other vesicular or weeping skin lesions are present and not securely covered. Chronic carriers need careful follow up, especially in a field where improvements in treatment constantly are becoming available.

More common causes of hepatitis in man

Pathogen	Transmission route
Hepatitis A virus	Orofaecal
Hepatitis B virus	Blood or sexual contact
Hepatitis C virus	Blood; sexual contact not common
Hepatitis D virus	Only in the presence of hepatitis B virus
Hepatitis E virus	Orofaecal

Less common causes of hepatitis in man

Pathogen	Transmission route
Epstein-Barr virus	Close contact
Cytomegalovirus	Close contact, blood
Toxoplasma gondii	Contact with cats, undercooked meat
Leptospira spp	Water

Rest is indicated until symptoms of hepatitis A subside, but a graded increase in exercise can be resumed before liver function tests return to normal

Chronic (post infection) fatigue syndrome

Chronic fatigue syndrome is discussed in detail in Chapter 10.

Skin infections

The skin is one of the main barriers to infection and infections of the skin are common in sportspeople.

Tetanus

Although rare, tetanus can be fatal, and all sportspeople vulnerable to "dirty" wounds should ensure their immunisation status is up to date. Infection is the result of infection by the organism *Clostridium tetani*. All wounds need careful consideration of whether a booster vaccination, human tetanus immunoglobulin, antibiotic, or combination, is indicated.

Viral infections

Molluscum contagiosum

Molluscum contagiosum is caused by a pox virus. The lesions are recognised by their characteristic umbilicated appearance. A number of strategies are available for treatment of molluscum: liquid nitrogen can be used locally on the lesions to good effect, an orange stick may be used to release the cheesy material from the lesion, and 25% podophyllin can be applied to the lesions once or twice a week.

Herpes simplex virus

In sports with close contact—for example, rugby and wrestling—an athlete who has herpes simplex may transmit the virus to a team mate or the opposition, leading to herpes gladiatorum or "scrumpox". Lesions on the fingers (herpetic whitlow) may be especially painful. Primary herpetic infections may give rise to a high fever, malaise, and prostration. Recurrences generally produce only a local problem, with characteristic clustered vesicles on an erythematous base. Herpes simplex infections may occasionally trigger more generalised erythema multiforme type lesions and, sometimes, full blown Stevens-Johnson syndrome, with mucous membrane involvement. The primary infection can be treated with oral antiviral drugs, such as valiciclovir or famciclovir. Patients with severe cases can be given antivirals parenterally.

Warts (verrucas)

Warts caused by the papova group of viruses may be a particular nuisance if they occur at important sites that interfere with sport. Warts will often disappear without treatment. Wart paints, a number of which contain salicylic acid, may be useful. Liquid nitrogen may be used in cryotherapy, and particularly troublesome warts can be curetted or removed surgically.

Bacterial infections

Streptococcal and staphylococcal infections

Streptococcal and staphylococcal infections of the skin are especially common in athletes. When the lower limb is involved, the portal of entry in sportspeople is often the location of athlete's foot. The diagnosis of a streptococcal or staphylococcal skin lesion is most often clinical. Wound swabs and blood culture may be helpful.

Streptococcal or staphylococcal infections may often spread rapidly and need to be treated urgently. The patient needs to be

---

Tetanus vaccination

Prophylaxis booster vaccination is needed:

- If the last immunisation was >10 years ago
- If the injured did not receive a full course of vaccination
- If the wound has an appreciable amount of devitalised tissue
- If the wound is a penetrating wound
- Where contact with soil or manure is evident
- In the presence of sepsis

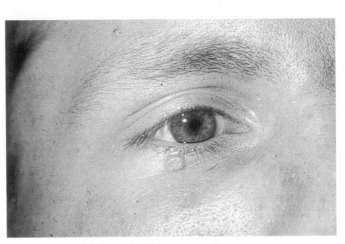

Raised pearly pink lesions of molluscum contagiosum

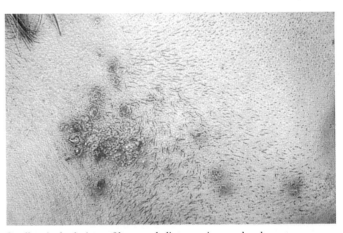

Small vesicular lesions of herpes gladiatorum in a rugby player

---

Signs that indicate systemic involvement of staphylococcal and streptococcal infections

- Clinical state of the patient
- High temperature
- High white cell count
- High erythrocyte sedimentation rate
- High levels of C reactive protein

isolated because of easy person to person spread. For localised lesions, treatment with oral penicillin and flucloxacillin in combination usually is adequate, although parenteral antibiotics may be needed, especially if the patient has signs of systemic involvement. For patients who are penicillin hypersensitive, a macrolide antibiotic, such as clindamycin, may be used. Meticulous care should be paid to hand washing to avoid local spread of infection.

Recurrent skin and ear infections

Some sportspeople become carriers of staphylococci, which often leads to recurrent infection, especially if the organisms gain access to small cuts and abrasions. Such carriers should take meticulous care when bathing and some may need to wash daily for 10 days with an antiseptic skin cleanser, such as povodine iodine (Betadine) or chlorhexidine (Hibiscrub), and apply an antibiotic nasal cream containing chlorhexidine (Naseptin) four times a day to the nostrils for 10 days to eradicate carriage of staphylococci.

Otitis externa can be a particular problem in swimmers and is easily diagnosed. The patient has a painful ear with discharge and characteristic erythematous findings on examination of the external auditory meatus. The infecting organisms may be a mixture of Gram positive and Gram negative bacteria, and treatment may need an antibiotic that is not used topically (such as neomycin or clioquinol). A local cream or ear drops that contain an antibiotic and steroid may be given for 7-10 days.

Fungal infections

Fungal infections are a particular problem in sites where sweat and moisture accumulate.

Tinea pedis (athlete's foot)

Athlete's foot characteristically presents as peeling of the skin, with fissuring and sometimes secondary infection, especially between the fourth and fifth toes. Often it is associated with blisters on the feet called podopomphylix. The most common infection is caused by *Trichophyton rubrum*, although infection from other fungi also occurs. The fissuring may be painful, but the most important complication of athlete's foot is secondary bacterial infection (ascending lymphangitis or cellulitis, or both).

Treatment involves meticulous washing and careful drying of the feet. An antifungal cream, such as co-trimazole, itraconazole or econazole, is effective. Oral terbinafine can be used if the lesions are in an inaccessible site or are extensive. Nail infections (tinea unguium) can be treated with terbinafine, which produces better results than griseofulvin and needs shorter treatment periods of six weeks to three months.

Tinea versicolor (Malassezia furfur)

Tinea versicolor produces areas of hypopigmented patches on the skin that are often scaly at the edges. Treatment consists of the application of selenium sulphide (Selsun) shampoo. Antifungal imidazole and terbinafine creams also are effective.

HIV

The risk of contracting HIV in sport related activities must be exceedingly small; to date, only one questionable case has been reported. The risk to sportspeople of HIV lies mainly in sexual intercourse. Sharing of razors and toothbrushes has a theoretical possibility of transmitting the virus and should be discouraged. At the same time, emphasis should be put on the fact that normal social contact and the sharing of changing facilities and swimming pools constitute no risk of infection.

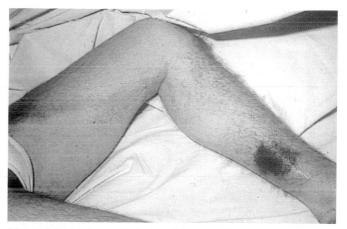

β haemolytic streptococcal infection of the leg, with tracking lymphangitis and inguinal lymphadenopathy

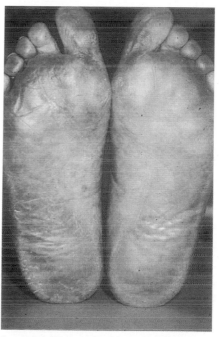

Severe involvement of feet in tinea pedis

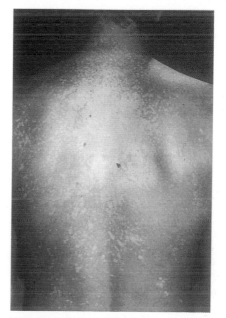

Hypopigmentation because of tinea (pityriasis) versicolor

Participants should be aware of the risk from injuries that result in bleeding from wounds; in all cases, such wounds should be covered or the player excluded from further participation. All participants, first aid workers, and accompanying sports staff should realise that, other than through sexual contact and other high risk practices, the risks of acquiring HIV infection in sport are very small, but general recommendations may apply.

Travel associated infections

Travellers' diarrhoea

Travellers' diarrhoea is by far the most common illness that afflicts travellers, and it varies with destination. Symptoms usually start on the third day abroad. Passage of blood or mucus, or both, implies bowel inflammation or ulceration and raises the likelihood of an invasive organism, such as *Shigella* spp. or *Entamoeba histolytica*, although *Salmonella* and *Campylobacter* can produce a similar picture. Giardiasis has a longer and usually more variable incubation period (often measured in weeks rather than days). *Cyclospora* as a cause of travellers' diarrhoea is a recent finding, especially in travellers who visit Nepal.

Dietary precautions, such as care in selecting well cooked food and consumption of only fresh fruit and vegetables that need peeling, are particularly important. Salads and uncooked shellfish are considered high risk. Only sterilised water should be consumed, including when brushing teeth and for ice in drinks. Because of their low pH (around 5.5) which kills organisms, bottled carbonated drinks are safe.

Prophylactic antimicrobials may be indicated in athletes who are staying abroad for less than two weeks and for whom peak performance is vital. In this case, the drug of choice would be ciprofloxacin (500 mg twice daily) as it covers most gastrointestinal pathogens. Reports are increasing, however, of quinolones induced tendonopathy in athletes. Co-trimoxazole (960 mg twice daily) and trimethoprim (200 mg twice daily) for five days are effective but more recently have been associated with development of haemolytic uraemic syndrome in people infected with *Escherichia coli* O157:H7. No antimicrobial thus is ideal, and their use in prophylaxis and proven gastroenteritis in athletes requires careful medical consideration. In addition, increasing resistance has been reported.

Treatment of travellers' diarrhoea is symptomatic. Milk should be avoided when symptoms are severe. Painful spasms may be treated with co-phenotrope (Lomotil) or loperamide (Imodium). These drugs should be used with caution and only for short periods of time, as nausea, vomiting, and sedation are associated with increasing doses, especially in the presence of renal impairment. They should not be used when diarrhoea is bloody, in which case medical advice should be sought.

Malarial chemoprophylaxis

Any person travelling to a malarial endemic area should be aware of the risk, avoid mosquito bites, take appropriate chemoprophylaxis, and seek immediate medical attention in the event of fever during and up to a year after travel. The spread of drug resistant *Plasmodium falciparum* malaria has complicated malarial chemoprophylaxis, as well as the awareness that some of the more effective (and now previously used) antimalarial combination drugs, such as sulfadoxine and pyrimethamine (Fansidar), pyrimethamine and dapsone (Maloprim), and amodiaquine, may have severe and sometimes fatal side effects. Further expert advice often may be needed. Drugs used most often for prophylaxis are mefloquine (Lariam), atovaquone and proguanil (Malarone), and doxycycline (Vibramycin).

Recommendations for handling injuries on sports field involving sportspeople who may be HIV positive

- Assume all casualties are HIV positive
- Wear gloves for all procedures that involve contact with blood or other body secretions
- Cover all cuts and abrasions where possible
- Wear protective glasses when blood may be splashed into face
- Wash skin immediately after contamination with blood or secretions
- Dispose of sharps safely; never attempt to resheathe needles
- Dispose of waste materials by burning
- Presoak contaminated clothes in hot (>70°C) soapy water for 30 minutes and then wash in a hot cycle washing machine; alternatively, soak clothes in household bleach (1 in 10 dilution) or solution containing sodium hypochlorite 2% (Milton solution) for 30 minutes
- All contaminated equipment or surfaces may be treated with bleach, as above
- Communal items in the first aid kit no longer have a place in the care of injured sportspeople (for example, bucket and sponge)
- No cases of HIV infection by mouth to mouth resuscitation have been recorded; however, simple devices that prevent direct contact between operator and patient are available to assist ventilation
- Where exposure to blood has occurred, further help should be sought with respect to counselling and the need for prophylactic antiviral drugs

---

Symptoms of giardiasis

- Persistent diarrhoea
- Flatulence
- Abdominal distension
- Lactose intolerance

Principal causes of travellers' diarrhoea

Bacteria
- Enterotoxigenic *Escherichia coli*
- *Shigella* spp.
- *Salmonella* spp.
- *Campylobacter jejuni*
- *Vibrio cholerae*
- Non-cholera vibrios, for example, *V. parahaemolyticus*

Viruses
- Rotavirus
- Small round viruses, for example, Norwalk agent

Protozoa
- *Giardia lamblia*
- *Entamoeba histolytica*
- *Cryptosporidium parvum*
- *Cyclospora cayetanensis*

Symptoms of travellers' diarrhoea

- Watery diarrhoea
- Cramps
- Nausea
- Vomiting
- Fever (in a few cases)
- Frank dysentery (sometimes)

If any doubt exists, specialist advice should be sought. Chemoprophylaxis should start at least a week before departure and continue while away and for four weeks after return (for atovaquone and proguanil, a day before entering an area with endemic malaria, while there and for seven days after return). The possibility of malaria should be considered in any person with a fever who is or has been in an area with endemic malaria, whether or not they have been taking antimalarial chemoprophylaxis. No current antimalarial drug can guarantee absolute protection.

Vaccination of travellers

Vaccination of travellers has become a routine, but it needs to be undertaken with consideration of the risks or benefits that are involved.

Further reading

- Goodman RA, Thacker SB, Solomon SL, Osterholm MT, Hughes JM. Infectious diseases in competitive sports. *JAMA* 1994;271:862-7
- Beck CK. Infectious diseases in sports. *Med Sci Sports Exerc* 2000;32:S431-8
- Mast EE, Goodman RA. Prevention of infectious disease transmission in sports. *Sports Med* 1997;24:1-7
- Sevier TL. Infectious disease in athletes. *Med Clin N Am* 1994;78:389-412
- Weber TS. Environmental and infectious conditions in sports. *Clin Sports Med* 2003;22:181-96
- Stacey A, Atkins B. Infectious diseases in rugby players: Incidence, treatment and prevention. *Sports Med* 2000;29:211-20
- Tobe K, Matsuura K, Ogura T, Tsuo Y, Iwasaki Y, Mizuno M, et al. Horizontal transmission of hepatitis B virus among players of an American football team. *Arch Intern Med* 2000;160:2541-5
- Bourliere M, Halfon P, Quentin Y, David P, Mengotti C, Portal I, et al. Covert transmission of hepatitis C virus during bloody fisticuffs. *Gastroenterology* 2000;119:507-11

Malarial chemoprophylaxis

Chemoprophylaxis	Area to be visited	Doses and comments
None	• North Africa (Morocco, Algeria, Tunisia, Libya, and tourist areas of Egypt) and tourist areas of South East Asia (Thailand, Philippines, Hong Kong, Singapore, Bali, China, and Vietnam)	
Chloroquine or proguanil (Paludrine)	• Middle East (including summer months in rural Egypt and Turkey), central America, and rural Mauritius	• Chloroquine 300 mg base (two tablets once per week)
Chloroquine and proguanil	• Indian subcontinent, Afghanistan, Iran and South America	• Proguanil 200 mg once per day • Doses as above
Mefloquine (Lariam)	• Sub-Saharan Africa, Papua New Guinea, Solomon Islands, and Vanuatu	• No longer recommended in sub-Saharan Africa • 250 mg (one tablet) once a week • Alternative to chloroquine and proguanil in areas of high risk • Possible increased risk of neuropsychiatric side effects
Doxycycline	• Mefloquine-resistant areas of southeast Asia (for example, Thai-Cambodian and Thai-Myanmar borders)	• 100 mg per day • Photosensitivity seen in 3% of patients who take this drug
Atovaquone and proguanil (Malarone)	• All malaria-endemic areas	• One tablet (250 mg atovaquone and 100 mg proguanil) daily • Useful for short visits—for example, Amazon basin, game parks, and multidrug resistant areas of southeast Asia

Vaccination of travellers

Vaccine	Dose	Comments
Polio*	• Three drops	• Primary course: three doses one month apart • Boost every 10 years
Tetanus (adsorbed tetanus toxin)	• 0.5 ml subcutaneously	• Primary course: three doses one month apart • Boost every 10 years up to a maximum of five vaccinations unless at special risk
Typhoid		
• Monovalent typhoid vaccine	• 0.5 ml intramuscularly for first dose, then 0.2 ml intradermally	• Primary course: two doses preferably a month and not less than 10 days apart • Boost every five years unless at special risk
• Live oral typhoid* vaccine strain Ty21A	• Three enteric coated capsules on alternate days	• Boost every three years unless at special risk
• Vi capsular polysaccharide typhoid vaccine	• 0.5 ml subcutaneously or intramuscularly once only	• Single boost every three years
Cholera	• 0.5 ml intramuscularly (first dose), then 0.1 ml intradermally	• Primary course: two doses preferably a month and not less than 10 days apart • Boosters every six months • Poor vaccine
Yellow fever*	• 0.5 ml subcutaneously	• Single injection from a recognised yellow fever centre with certificate (valid 10 days after vaccination for 10 years)
Hepatitis A (human diploid cell)	• 1 ml intramuscularly	• Primary course: a single dose (>1440 ELISA units of hepatitis A protein). For immunity years, booster at 6-12 months
Hepatitis B	• 1 ml intramuscularly	• Primary course: 0, 1, and 6 months • One booster at 3-5 years
Rabies (human diploid cell vaccine)	• 1 ml intramuscularly or 0.1 ml intradermally**	• Primary course: three doses one month apart • Booster every 2-3 years

*Indicates live vaccine
**Not standard recommendation, but probably as effective, cheaper and less likely to cause side effects

10   Unexplained underperformance syndrome (overtraining syndrome)

Richard Budgett

Many athletes have a week or two of relative underperformance at times of hard training. Sometimes this underperformance, normally accompanied by fatigue, persists for more than two weeks despite adequate rest.

The first duty of the doctor is to exclude underlying illness with an appropriate history and examination. A full blood count with measurement of iron stores and thyroid function may identify unexpected causes, otherwise routine blood screening rarely is helpful. In most underperforming (and normally fatigued) athletes, no cause is found and they are diagnosed as having unexplained underperformance syndrome.

Symptoms

Underperforming athletes present with fatigue, heavy muscles, and depression. Direct questioning reveals sleep disturbance with difficulty getting to sleep, nightmares, waking in the night, or prolonged sleep but waking unrefreshed. Other symptoms are loss of motivation, energy, competitive drive, and libido; altered mood state profiles; increased anxiety and irritability; loss of appetite with weight loss; increased lightheadedness (postural hypotension); and a high resting pulse rate. Some athletes have frequent minor infections, breaking down with an upper respiratory tract infection every 3-4 weeks.

Distinguishing symptoms

Distinguishing unexplained underperformance syndrome from normal training fatigue (over-reaching) is difficult and can only be done once an athlete has failed to recover. Many athletes will be fatigued, irritable, anxious, and depressed, with a high resting pulse rate and minor infections but will nevertheless recover quickly once the training has been reduced—certainly within two weeks. Athletes have to train hard to improve and the challenge for doctors and sports scientists is to develop reliable measures of recovery so that athletes can train as hard as possible but not so hard that they break down for many weeks with unexplained underperformance syndrome.

Training history

Often an athlete has a history of an increase or change in training. Many athletes break down when they switch from low intensity winter training to high intensity summer training with intensive interval work. The stress of competition and selection pressures also may contribute. Athletes usually can keep up with the beginning of a race but describe an inability to lift the pace or sprint for the line.

One swimmer broke the British record and decided to cut his rest day to train for seven days a week instead of six days. He broke down after several months and took many weeks to recover. Another swimmer increased his training to eight hours a day. For four months, his performance improved but then he started to fail to recover from training. He took months to recover fully.

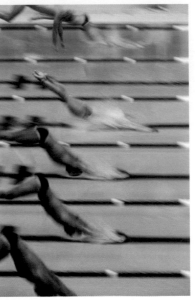

Unexplained underperformance syndrome occurs in up to 10% of elite endurance athletes per year, but the problem is not confined to Olympic athletes: 10% of collegiate swimmers in the United States are described as "burning out" each year

Definitions
- Over-reaching—hard training with adequate recovery
- Overtraining—hard training without adequate recovery
- Unexplained underperformance syndrome—unexplained underperformance for at least two weeks despite adequate rest

Symptoms of unexplained underperformance syndrome
- Underperformance
- Depression with loss of motivation, competitive drive and libido
- Increased anxiety and irritability
- Sleep disturbance
- Loss of appetite and weight
- Fatigue
- Frequent minor infections particularly of the upper respiratory tract
- Raised resting pulse rate
- Increased symptoms of postural hypotension

Other names for unexplained underperformance syndrome
- Overtraining syndrome
- Chronic fatigue in athletes
- Sports fatigue syndrome
- Burnout
- Staleness
- Under-recovery syndrome

Precipitating factors of unexplained underperformance syndrome
- Training, especially interval training or sudden increase in training
- Stress of competition
- Other stresses such as:
  Glycogen depletion
  Dehydration
  Other illness or injury
  Other psychological stress of life events—for example, exams, moving house, or relationship problems

Nevertheless, athletes rarely break down after less than two weeks of hard training (as in a typical training camp), as long as they rest and allow themselves to recover afterwards. This is what happens with normal tapering.

In some sports, training is heavy and monotonous and lacks much periodisation (cyclical variation of training). This makes it more difficult to recover from exercise. Large volumes of training are generally well tolerated, however, as long as the intensity is low enough.

Other stresses

For most athletes, training is no different to that of other athletes or that of previous years. Adequate recovery is likely to be the critical factor. Stresses such as exams and other life events, glycogen depletion because of poor diet, and dehydration will reduce the ability to recover or respond to heavy training.

One rower moved 600 miles to train with a new coach, giving up her career and leaving friends and family behind. After three months, she developed unexplained underperformance syndrome despite being used to the level of training and commitment needed. She recovered over two months with an appropriate regeneration programme.

Signs

Signs are inconsistent and generally unhelpful in making a diagnosis because they vary greatly between individuals. Commonly reported signs are increased postural drop in blood pressure and postural rise in heart rate. A reduction in all measures of performance is seen. Changes in heart rate variability and increased resting heart rate and increased vulnerability to minor infections may occur.

Investigation

History and examination should guide doctors in deciding whether further investigations might be helpful. Often it is difficult to persuade athletes and coaches of a diagnosis of unexplained underperformance syndrome, so some basic screening may be needed to confirm no undiagnosed illness is present. Some serious diseases, such as viral myocarditis or cardiac abnormalities, have presented as unexplained underperformance syndrome, but this is very rare. Prolonged glycogen depletion because of disordered eating (or even eating disorders such as anorexia or bulimia) is a more common cause of fatigue and underperformance. Allergic rhinitis and atopy may present as recurrent upper respiratory tract infections.

Laboratory tests
Laboratory tests are occasionally helpful but cannot be used to make a diagnosis of unexplained underperformance syndrome.

Full blood count
Haemoglobin concentrations and packed cell volume decrease as a normal response to heavy training and athletes reported anaemia is often physiological caused by haemodilution and does not affect performance.

Iron stores
Low serum ferritin concentrations, which reflect iron stores, are now accepted to cause fatigue in the absence of anaemia. Serum ferritin levels may be affected by concurrent illness. Most menstruating endurance athletes have ferritin levels of less than 30 μl which may contribute to fatigue, and

---

Signs of over-reaching (which is normal if athletes recover quickly)
- High serum creatine kinase concentration
- Low ratio of serum testosterone to cortisol concentrations
- Falls in muscle glycogen concentration
- Raised resting heart rate
- Mood deterioration
- Changes in heart rate variability
- Increased vulnerability to minor infections

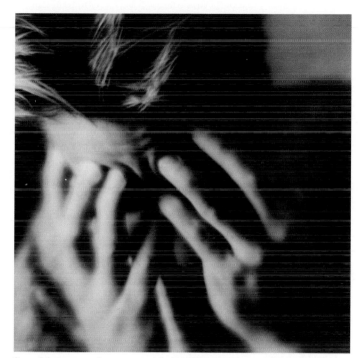

Stressful events, such as exams, relationship problems, moving house, or homesickness, will reduce an athlete's ability to recover or respond to heavy training

---

Exclusion of other causes of chronic fatigue

History
- Enquire about:
  Infection
  Wheeze
  Eating disorders
  Chest pain
  Shortness of breath on exercise

Examination
- To exclude a medical cause

Investigations
- Depend on clinical possibilities but may include:
  Laboratory tests
  Lung function
  Cardiac tests

Laboratory tests rarely help in the diagnosis of chronic fatigue

---

Overtraining may cause immunosuppression through:
- High serum cortisol concentrations
- Low serum glutamine concentrations
- Low salivary immunoglobulin A concentrations and saliva volume
- Low T helper to T suppressor cell ratios

this is particularly important if they are considering altitude training.

Viruses

Viral titres may be shown to be high or the Paul-Bunnell test may be positive, which strongly suggests glandular fever. Nevertheless, identification of a specific virus does not change the management and is therefore of limited value.

Trace elements and vitamins

No link has been shown between vitamins, trace elements, and unexplained underperformance syndrome. The widespread use of supplements by athletes does not seem to offer any protection from fatigue and underperformance, and it should be discouraged because of the risk of contamination.

Prevention and early detection

Although unexplained underperformance syndrome, by definition, is unexplained, hard training with inadequate recovery is a typical preceding picture.

Athletes can tolerate different levels of training and competition stress. Excessive training for one may be insufficient training for another. Each athlete's tolerance level will also change through the season, so training must be individualised and varied and should be reduced at times of stresses such as exams. Unfortunately, athletes are exhausted most of the time, unless they are tapering for a competition, so it is difficult for them to differentiate early unexplained underperformance syndrome from over-reaching. Investigators have tried to identify strategies for early detection.

Heart rate

A persistent rise in early morning heart rate, despite rest, is non-specific but does provide objective evidence that something is wrong. Heart rate variability has been used for decades by the Eastern bloc to monitor the training status of athletes. Changes in the balance of the activity of the sympathetic and parasympathetic nervous systems occur with hard training and then recovery (with high parasympathetic drive after successful tapering). This may be reflected in heart rate variability, which gives an objective guide to the extent of recovery. Unfortunately, changes in athletes with unexplained underperformance syndrome are very variable, so heart rate variability cannot be used to make a reliable diagnosis. Heart rate variability seems to change unpredictably as athletes go through fatigue, exhaustion, detraining, and recovery. Nevertheless, a reliable pattern might be obtained if individual athletes are followed.

Other factors

Performance should be monitored carefully, and underperformance after a taper is probably most important. Serial measurements of blood concentrations of haemoglobin and creatine kinase are unlikely to help.

Prevention requires good diet, full hydration, and rest between training sessions. Coaches and athletes must realise that sportspeople with full time jobs and other commitments will not recover as quickly as those who can relax after training. Periodisation of training should ensure recovery. No reliable objective test yet predicts which athletes will break down after a period of hard training.

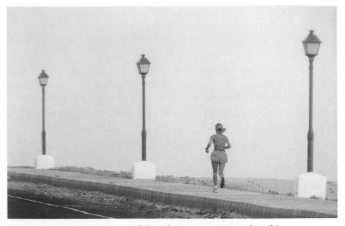

Many sports and exercise medicine doctors recommend oral iron (often a liquid preparation, as this seems to be better tolerated) and vitamin C to help absorption for most female endurance athletes who are menstruating

> Dietary advice should be sought by all athletes, and they must be given strong reassurance that a varied diet with sufficient calories negates the need for supplements.

> In American college swimmers, a 10% incidence of burn out was reduced to zero by daily mood monitoring with a profile of mood state questionnaire, reducing training whenever mood deteriorated, and increasing it when mood improved

Early detection of unexplained underperformance syndrome is difficult, but individual monitoring may help

- Performance
- Mood state
- Resting heart rate
- Heart rate variability
- Glutamine to glutamate ratio

> In some athletes, immune parameters may change with low levels of serum glutamine and changes in levels of salivary immunoglobulin A and serum cortisol

Management

Sports medicine doctors must work with coach and athlete to agree a recovery programme. The most important task is to persuade coach and athlete of the diagnosis and that prolonged recovery is needed. Athletes will benefit from a multidisciplinary approach and should see a sports dietician and sports psychologist if available. Physiologists can also help by setting training levels. During this time, rest and regeneration strategies are essential to recovery.

Therapeutic exercise

Evidence shows that a very low level of exercise will help patients with chronic fatigue syndrome recover. Athletes with unexplained underperformance syndrome show improvement in performance and mood state with five weeks of relative rest. Athletes are advised to exercise aerobically at a level well below anaerobic threshold for a few minutes each day and to slowly build this up over many weeks. The starting level and speed of increase in training volume will depend on the clinical picture and rate of improvement. Recovery generally takes 6-12 weeks. Unless held strictly to a recovery programme, many make the mistake of trying to do a normal training session when feeling a little better, suffering from severe fatigue for several days before partially recovering and doing it again. Cross training (playing another sport) may be the only way to avoid the tendency to increase the intensity too fast. Once athletes can tolerate 20 minutes of light exercise each day, introduction of short sprints of less than 10 seconds with at least three minutes recovery between each sprint is useful.

If an athlete is depressed, evidence shows that a graded exercise programme will not be effective unless the depression is treated (with an antidepressant and psychological intervention). Antidepressants also may be helpful in mildly depressed athletes with disturbed sleep.

Athletes often are surprised at the performance they can produce after 12 weeks of extremely light exercise. Care must then be taken not to increase training too fast. When returning to normal training, consideration of alternate hard and light days is helpful. As athletes return to full training, they are advised to train hard but to rest and recover completely at least once a week to benefit from all their hard work.

Management of unexplained underperformance syndrome

- Very light exercise
- Relaxation strategies and rest
- Convince coach and athlete of the diagnosis
- Strong reassurance that the prognosis is good
- Very short sprints with long rests as condition improves

Athletes with unexplained underperformance syndrome compared with patients with chronic fatigue syndrome

- Primary presenting complaint is underperformance—an objective measure of the condition
- Athletes present earlier, are less severely affected, and recover more quickly
- Main stresses in lives are exercise and competition, which can be controlled
- Main problem in rehabilitation is to hold athletes back rather than having to encourage appropriate exercise

---

Typical rehabilitation programme

Week	Programme
1	20 minutes of light exercise per day at pulse rate of 120 7 × 10 second sprints or weights three times a week
2	30 minutes of light exercise, including 10 × 10 seconds sprint
3	40 minutes of light exercise, including 10 × 10 seconds sprint
4	50 minutes of light exercise, including 10 × 10 seconds sprint
5	60 minutes of light exercise, including 10 × 10 seconds sprint
6	60 minutes of light exercise, including 2 × 2 minutes normal intensity
6-10	Build up normal intensity in 60 minutes to full 60 minutes at normal intensity
10-12	Add second session Increase to normal training

11 Female athlete triad

Karen Birch

The "female athlete triad" long has been recognised as a syndrome that has the potential to affect female athletes and consists of three interrelated disorders:

- Osteoporosis
- Disordered eating
- Menstrual disorders.

The potential impact of each of, and the combination of, these disorders to the athlete is detrimental to performance and to health. Certainly, the increased risk of infertility, stress fractures, eating disorders, and osteoporosis in later life is a high price to pay for involvement in an essentially healthy activity. This is especially true, as many of these factors can be prevented with careful management.

Why are the three corners of the triad interrelated?

The three corners of the triad are interrrelated through psychological and physiological mechanisms. The psychological pressures to perform to an optimal standard, and thus often a perceived requirement to maintain a low body mass, result in a high volume of training. The high volume of training and low kilocaloric intake, in addition to stress hormones produced by psychological stress, may lead to a physiological alteration in the endocrinological control of the menstrual cycle, which may ultimately lead to the athlete becoming amenorrhoeic (loss of cycle). The consequence of being amenorrhoeic is a dysfunction of the hypothalamus and pituitary, which leads to decreased production of oestrogen. This hormone has a huge role to play in maintaining adequate bone mineral density, and a hypo-oestrogenic state (low oestrogen) thus is associated with low bone mineral density and an increased risk of osteoporosis.

Menstrual disorders

The normal regular, healthy menstrual cycle (eumenorrhoea) is about 26-35 days in length, is controlled by the hypothalamus and pituitary glands, and is divided simplistically into two phases by the occurrence mid-cycle of ovulation. The first half of the cycle is the follicular phase and the second half the luteal phase. The follicular phase is characterised by gradually increasing levels of oestrogen produced primarily by the ovaries, while the luteal phase is characterised by high concentrations of oestrogen and progesterone. In addition, some oestrogen is synthesised in adipose tissue cells.

Menstrual cycle disturbances can progress from luteal phase defects to anovulation (no ovulation) and then to oligomenorrhoea (irregular cycles) and amenorrhoea. The diagnosis of luteal phase defects includes criteria such as a luteal phase less than 10 days long, inadequate progesterone concentration, ultrasound measurement of preovulatory follicle diameter, and endometrial biopsy.

Causes in athletes

Causes of menstrual disorders are multiple and not completely understood. Pulsatile release of luteinising hormone is decreased, which leads initially to luteal phase defects. In addition, compared with sedentary women, women with luteal phase defects and amenorrhoea have higher levels of growth hormone and cortisol and lower levels of leptin, insulin, and

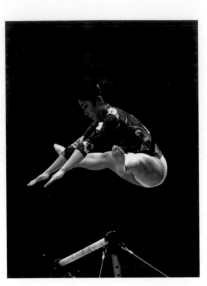

The effect of one or more of the disorders of the female athlete triad can affect performance and health but this can be prevented with good management

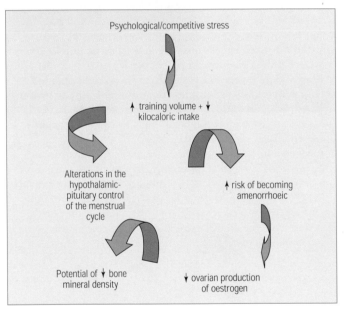

The corners of the female athlete triad (osteoporosis, disordered eating, and menstrual disorders) are interrelated through psychological and physiological mechanisms

Prevalence of amenorrhoea
- Population—5%
- Athletes—1-44% (luteal phase defects 79%)

Legend has it low levels of body fat in female athletes and lack of production of peripherally produced oestrogen disrupts the menstrual cycle to cause luteal phase defects and amenorrhoea. This is not the case

Luteal phase defects may be less obvious than amenorrhoea in athletes, but the clinical consequences are serious

triiodothyronine. These hormones are related to metabolism, and thus to nutritional and metabolic status. If energy availability is low over a period of time, as indicated by these hormones, the menstrual cycle is temporarily "switched off" or suppressed as a potential method of conserving energy.

> The potential cause of menstrual disturbances in women athletes is not training per se but being in a negative energy balance. Adequate nutritional intake to match the requirements of training thus is essential

Eating disorder or disordered eating?

Some female athletes do suffer from a classic eating disorder, potentially driven by a need to maintain a low body mass for performance. Anorexia, however, has very specific clinical diagnostic criteria, and athletes may or may not satisfy the criteria that indicate a disturbance in how they experience body weight or shape. The term "anorexia athletica" has been used in research literature to distinguish between pathological anorexia and eating disorders associated with training and sports performance. The criteria for this include perfectionism, compulsiveness, competitiveness, high self-motivation, menstrual disturbances, and at least one unhealthy method of weight control (fasting, vomiting, use of diet pills, laxatives, or diuretics). In reality, athletes in this category will show signs of disordered eating, as opposed to an eating disorder, and clinical observations indicate a prevalence of 15-60% for disordered eating, with 50% of these women compulsively overexercising. This will obviously lead to a decreased kilocaloric intake and thus a negative energy balance.

> Energy balance = energy in   energy out
>
> Women athletes who attempt to keep body mass low tend to reduce their energy intake but continue to train hard, keeping the energy output very high. This leads to a lowered energy availability

Osteoporosis or osteopenia?

Osteoporosis is defined as a bone mineral density more than 2.5 standard deviations below the average for young adults and is associated with a reduction in bone mass with no alteration in the mineralisation of bone tissue. Bone tissue responds well to mechanical stress, and thus exercise, alongside nutrition, is essential in the teenage years for attainment of peak bone mass. For women with low energy availability and low oestrogen concentrations, however, the risk of becoming osteoporotic is enhanced. Oestrogen protects the skeleton from bone resorption, while deficiencies in calcium, vitamin D, and other bonetrophic substances from adequate nutritional intake also lead to increased bone resorption. Indeed, a reduced long term risk of osteoporosis seems to be related to attaining a good peak bone mineral density in early life and to the lifelong exposure to oestrogen. Thus, long periods of amenorrhoea may increase the long term risk of osteoporosis.

A recent paper called for a change in the criteria for the female athlete triad, as the occurrence of osteoporosis in female athletes is quite small.[1] Indeed, Rutherford et al. reported a 13% prevalence of osteoporosis in amenorrhoeic triathletes and distance runners but a 40% prevalence of osteopenia.[2] Osteopenia is defined as a bone mineral density score between 1 and 2.5 standard deviations below the average of young adults and is characterised by decreased calcification of bone. Certainly, any reduction in bone mineral density, regardless of size, should be deemed negative for the athlete, and thus the inclusion of osteopenia in the triad definitely is warranted, as both conditions increase the risk of stress fracture.

> A low percentage of body fat is associated with negative energy balance. Thus, a low percentage of body fat should be seen as a signal that disordered eating and menstrual disturbances may be present

Effects of menstrual disturbances on bone mineral density

Studies that compare eumenorrhoeic and amenorrhoeic athletes have consistently shown a lower bone mineral density in amenorrhoeic athletes. Amenorrhoeic runners have been reported to have lower bone mineral density at the spine (−5%), hip (−6%), and whole body (−3%) than eumenorrhoeic runners. Furthermore, eumenorrhoeic runners with disordered eating patterns have lower bone mineral density at the spine

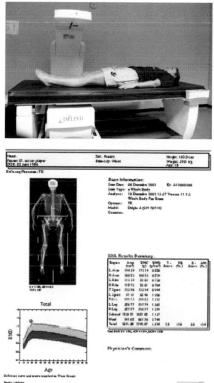

Athlete having a bone scan and print out of results

(−11%), hip (−5%), and whole body (−5%) than eumenorrhoeic runners without disordered eating. Athletes with less severe menstrual disruption have intermediate bone densities. The bone mineral density of the femur in amenorrhoeic athletes is closer to that of sedentary controls than that in the spine. This suggests that participation in regular running (or weight bearing activity) can offset bone loss because of menstrual disturbances.

> Athletes with menstrual disturbances can increase bone mineral density with weight bearing exercise or treatment on reversal of the menstrual disturbance. Bone mineral density, however, will never return to what it may have been if the athlete had remained eumenorrhoeic. If trabeculae bone is lost during long term amenorrhoea, reversal of bone mineral density may be impossible

Evaluation of athletes

The American College of Sports Medicine produced an *Evaluation of the female athlete triad: a guide to physicians.* This guide details the criteria for assessing disordered eating, the symptoms of starvation and purging, which laboratory tests are indicated, which factors are required to conduct a menstrual, exercise, family, psychological, and nutritional history, and any further recommended tests. The "SCOFF" questionnaire may be used to assess eating disorders.

Treatment of female athlete triad

Prevention is likely to yield better benefits than treatment, but prevention in athletes is made difficult by the nature of the game. Athletes will resist increasing body weight, decreasing training loads, and consumption of the oral contraceptive pill (because of worries about weight gain, breast tenderness, and mood changes). In addition, an admission of menstrual problems and disordered eating or eating disorders will also prove difficult for female athletes. In consultation with the athlete, these points should be kept firmly in mind.

Eating disorders
The treatment of true eating disorders should only be undertaken by qualified personnel on an inpatient or outpatient basis. The treatment plan will vary for each individual based on psychology and environment, but a number of common sense guidelines exist for people who work with women athletes.

The ultimate goal is to increase the nutritional status of the woman. This will reverse many of the symptoms associated with disordered eating (for example, bloating, constipation, fatigue, lanugo, dry skin, and so on—although not loss of enamel from teeth), reverse menstrual disorders, and help reduce the risk of osteopenia or osteoporosis. Of course, many of these changes will ultimately increase muscle strength, decrease the risk of injury, and thus increase training and sports performance.

Menstrual disturbances
Once disturbances have been established as non-pathological (the athlete should be medically assessed), the treatment is based on training load and nutritional intake. Athletes will benefit from decreased training intensities or durations of 10%; they then should look to increase kilocaloric intake by initially small amounts.

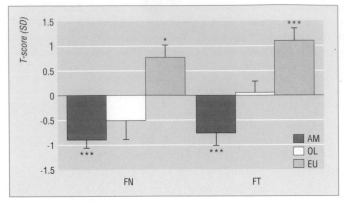

Bone mineral density of the proximal femur of 50 endurance trained female runners compared with the young peak bone mass according to a standard reference range (Hologic Inc). This is known as the T score and is expressed in standard deviations above or below the mean. This chart shows the approximate linear relationship between number of menstrual cycles per year and bone density. (AM = amenorrhoeic (0-3 cycles a year), OL = oligomenorrhoeic (4-10 cycles per year), EU = eumenorrhoeic (11-13 cycles per year), FN = neck of femur, FT = trochanteric region of proximal femur. T test compares each group with the Hologic range (*p < 0.02, **p < 0.01, ***p < 0.001)

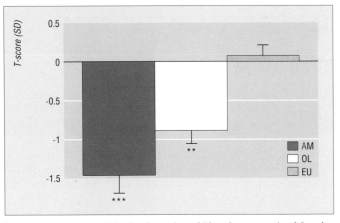

Bone mineral density of the lumbar spine of 50 endurance trained female runners compared with the young peak bone mass according to a standard reference range (Hologic Inc). This is known as the T score and is expressed in standard deviations above or below the mean. This chart shows the approximate linear relationship between number of menstrual cycles per year and bone density. (AM = amenorrhoeic (0-3 cycles a year), OL = oligomenorrhoeic (4-10 cycles per year), EU = eumenorrhoeic (11-13 cycles per year). T test compares each group with the Hologic range (*p < 0.02, **p < 0.01, ***p < 0.001)

> All individuals and agencies involved with female athletes need to be made fully aware of the potential causes, mechanisms, and long term risks of the female athlete triad. In addition, women athletes, their parents, and medical staff should be apprised of the triad and its pitfalls. The management of the athlete, however, is most imperative

> It is important to highlight that energy balance is matching kilocaloric intake and expenditure and that when this is achieved, no increase in body weight will be seen but maintenance of muscle mass will increase performance

Menstrual disturbances and decreased bone mineral density
Treatment is reliant on oestrogen replacement. Oestrogen replacement can be provided with the oral contraceptive pill, although progesterone only pills and the mini pill should be avoided. If the athlete agrees to take the pill, they should understand that it does not correct the underlying problem. If menses (bleeding) is not desired, the practitioner can sometimes provide monophasic pills in which the placebo week is missing. This, however, should only be a short term approach. Hormone replacement therapy, as provided for postmenopausal women, has only been successful in a few studies. Hormone replacement therapy with unopposed oestrogens should be avoided and should not be used for long periods.

Other treatments recommended for bone loss are specific oestrogen receptor modulators, intranasal calcitonin, and biphosphonates. These products are used primarily in older women, and little is known about their effects on bone mineral density in amenorrhoeic women. Calcium intake should be increased to 1500-2000 mg a day, and calcium should be taken alongside vitamin D. Calcium does not increase bone mineral density but may aid in preventing further decreases.

1 Khan K, Liu-Ambrose T, Sran M, Ashe M, Donaldson M, Wark J. New criteria for female athlete triad syndrome? *Br J Sports Med* 2002;36:10-3
2 Rutherford O. Spine and total body mineral density in amenorrheic endurance athletes. *J App Physiol* 1993;74:2904-8

Useful organisations

- American College of Sports Medicine, 401 West Michigan Street, Indianapolis, IN 46202-3233, USA (www.acsm.org)
- National Osteoporosis Society, Camerton, Bath BA2 0PJ (www.nos.org.uk)

> **Treatment of female athlete triad is based on behavioural change and reversal of chronic energy deficiency**

Further reading

- American College of Sports Medicine. Position stand on the female athlete triad. *Med Sci Sports Exercise* 1997;29:1-9
- De Souza MJ. Menstrual disturbances in athletes: A focus on luteal phase defects. *Med Sci Sports Exercise* 2003;35:1553-63
- Drinkwater B. *Women in sport. The encyclopaedia of sports medicine.* Blackwell Science, Oxford, 2000
- Loucks A, Vurdun M, Heath E. Low energy availability, not stress of exercise, alters LH pulsatility in exercising women. *J App Physiol* 1998;84:37-46
- Morgan JF, Reid F, Lacey JH. The SCOFF questionnaire: assessment of a new screening tool for eating disorders. *BMJ* 1999;319:1467-8

The graphs of bone mineral density in female athletes are adapted from Gibson JH, Mitchell A, Harries M, Reeve J. Nutritional and exercise related determinants of bone density in elite female runners. *Osteoporosis Int* 2004;15:611-8. The photo of the gymnast is reproduced with permission from Getty Images Ltd.

12 The athlete's heart and sudden cardiac death

Gregory P Whyte, Sanjay Sharma, Jayesh Makan, Nigel Stephens, William J McKenna

A large heart and slow heart rate are well recognised features of athletes' hearts. This article looks at the structure and function of the athlete's heart and the phenomenon of sudden cardiac death in athletes.

Athlete's heart

Adaptation of the human heart to physical training has been the focus of study for doctors and sports scientists since the late nineteenth century. Regular systematic physical training is associated with a number of unique structural and functional adaptations that enhance cardiac output during exercise. Ventricular hypertrophy, increase in cardiac chamber size, and enhanced ventricular filling in diastole enable an increased stroke volume at rest and during exercise. Athletes also have reduced resting heart rates, possibly because of the functional effect of an increased stroke volume. A large heart and slow heart rate are features of athletes' hearts and manifest as a displaced and forceful cardiac apical impulse on physical examination, large QRS complexes, sinus bradycardia, first and second degree heart block on a 12 lead electrocardiogram, and a high cardiothoracic ratio on plain chest radiographs.[1]

Cardiac dimensions in highly trained athletes

Training induced adaptations in cardiac structure traditionally have been divided into two main types depending on the specific nature of the haemodynamic load placed on the heart. Exercise associated with a sustained increase in preload (endurance training) is associated with left ventricular cavity dilatation and minor increases in wall thickness. In contrast, exercise associated with a predominant increase in afterload (strength training) is associated with an increased left ventricular wall thickness and relatively normal sized left ventricular cavity dimension. Limited evidence exists, however, for this compartmentalisation of cardiac adaptation to training because of the variety of training methods used in sport. In most athletes, cardiac adaptations exhibited tend to reflect a combination of responses to increased preload and afterload.

Studies of cardiac dimensions in athletes show large overlap with matched non-athletic controls. In absolute terms, cardiac dimensions in athletes are very slightly increased compared with non-athletes. Although the difference is small, it does reach statistical significance and amounts to a 15-20% larger left ventricular wall thickness and 10% larger left ventricular cavity compared with non-athletes. The modest increases in left ventricular wall thickness and left ventricular cavity size result in a marked increase in left ventricular mass.[4]

Most athletes have cardiac dimensions within normal limits for the general population—that is, a left ventricular wall thickness <12 mm and left ventricular cavity size <55 mm. A proportion of athletes, however, have a left ventricular wall thickness, and more commonly a left ventricular cavity size, that exceeds predicted normal limits. In this group of athletes, cardiac dimensions may be similar to those seen in patients with morphologically mild hypertrophic and dilated cardiomyopathy respectively.[2,5,6]

Upper normal limits for left ventricular wall thickness have been identified in adult and adolescent athletes.[2,5,6] In men and women athletes, wall thickness values >14 mm and >12 mm, respectively, warrant further investigation to exclude

Cardiac adaptations in an athlete

- Training results in increased left ventricular muscle mass
- The largest hearts are seen in athletes who participate in events that need a combination of endurance and strength and power
- Adaptations are similar between men and women and junior and senior athletes; however, men have larger hearts than women and seniors larger hearts than juniors
- Cardiac enlargement is reversible in athletes
- Diastolic and systolic function are normal or enhanced in athletes
- Upper normal limits of left ventricular wall thickness for men and women are 14 mm and 12 mm, respectively. Values in excess of these should indicate further examination

The combined strength and endurance training used in certain sports, such as rowing, cycling, canoeing, triathlon, swimming, and rugby, may be associated with substantial increases in left ventricular wall thickness and left ventricular cavity size[2,3]

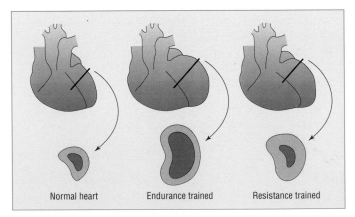

Left ventricular adaptation to physical training

Normal heart   Endurance trained   Resistance trained

Differentiation between physiological cardiac enlargement (athlete's heart) and cardiomyopathy is crucial when the fact that cardiomyopathies are the most common cause of exercise related sudden death is considered

hypertrophic cardiomyopathy. In adolescent athletes, left ventricular wall thickness >12 mm should also raise the suspicion of hypertrophic cardiomyopathy.

Cardiac function

Normal or enhanced indices of left ventricular systolic and diastolic function are seen in the athlete's hearts despite considerable increases in left ventricular mass.

Electrocardiograms

Bradycardia, sinus arrhythmia, voltage criteria for left ventricular enlargement, and early repolarisation changes such as tall T waves and concave ST segment elevations are common electrocardiographic manifestations of athlete's heart. Incomplete right bundle branch block (possibly reflecting right ventricular enlargement) also is relatively common. First degree heart block and Mobitz type I second degree atrioventricular block also are recognised findings; however, higher degrees of atrioventricular block are rare. Minor T wave inversions are seen and are usually confined to the right chest leads (V1, V2, and V3), but ST segment depression or deep (> 0.3 mV) T waves are uncommon. Pathological Q waves and left bundle branch block are not features of the athlete's heart.

Sudden cardiac death

A very small but significant number of athletes die suddenly. Most deaths occur during or immediately after exercise and are rarely preceded by prodromal symptoms indicative of cardiovascular disease. The precise incidence of sudden cardiac death in young athletes is unknown; however, such tragedies are highly publicised, which leads to major concern in the general population, which perceives athletes as the healthiest proportion of the population.

Some 80% of non-traumatic sudden deaths in young athletes result from inherited structural and functional cardiovascular abnormalities. Hypertrophic cardiomyopathy accounts for about one third of all sudden cardiac deaths. It is a disorder of the sarcomeric contractile protein and is characterised by left ventricular hypertrophy, a small left ventricular cavity, impaired myocardial relaxation, and a propensity to fatal ventricular arrhythmias. The prevalence of hypertrophic cardiomyopathy is 1 in 500. Most deaths in hypertrophic cardiomyopathy occur during or immediately after exercise. Death is more common in males.

Other inherited causes include arrhythmogenic right ventricular cardiomyopathy, coronary artery anomalies, premature coronary artery disease, ion channelopathies including long QT and Brugada's syndrome, Marfan's syndrome, mitral valve prolapse, and Wolf-Parkinson-White syndrome. Evidence suggests that systematic cardiovascular screening may be effective in identifying people with conditions predisposing to sudden cardiac death during sport.[7] The authors recommend detailed screening in individuals with symptoms suggestive of cardiac disease and those with a family history of premature sudden cardiac death (aged <40 years). Investigations should include resting electrocardiogram, two dimensional echocardiography, integrated cardiopulmonary stress test, and a 24 hour electrocardiogram. A small group of athletes may need more invasive investigations, such as cardiac catheterisation and electrophysiological studies.

Commotio cordis

Another mechanism for sudden cardiac death in athletes who are free of cardiac disease is blunt chest impact produced by a projectile or by collision with another athlete (commotio cordis).

Common and uncommon results from resting 12 lead electrocardiograms in junior elite athletes

Common	Uncommon
• Sinus bradycardia or arrhythmia	
• First degree atrioventricular block	• Second (Mobitz II and advanced) and third atrioventricular block
• QT and QRS elongation	• QT > 0.44 ms
• Left ventricular hypertrophy (Sokolow-Lyon)	• Left ventricular hypertrophy (Romhilt Estes) in women
• Left atrial or right atrial enlargement	
• ST segment elevation	• ST depression in any lead
• Tall T waves	• Deep T wave inversion
• Partial right bundle branch block	• Minor T wave inversion (>16 years)

Causes of sudden cardiac death

Common	Uncommon
• Hypertrophic cardiomyopathy*	• Myocarditis
• Coronary artery anomalies	• Coronary artery disease
• Arrhythmogenic right ventricular cardiomyopathy†	• Long QT or Brugada's syndrome
	• Marfan's syndrome
	• Mitral valve prolapse
	• Wolf-Parkinson-White syndrome
	• Aortic stenosis

*Most common cause of exercise related sudden cardiac death
†Most common cause of exercise related sudden cardiac death in northern Italy

---

Characteristics of hypertrophic cardiomyopathy

• Left ventricular hypertrophy
• Small left ventricular cavity
• Impaired myocardial relaxation
• Propensity to fatal ventricular arrhythmias

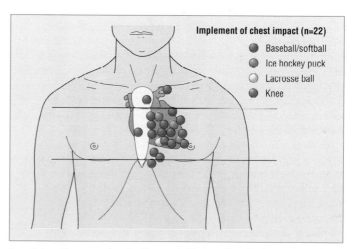

Locations of impact points leading to sudden cardiac death in 22 victims of commotio cordis. Adapted from Maron BJ. *Cardiac Electrophys Rev* 2002;6.100-3

Three determinants of commotio cordis have been identified:

- Relatively low energy chest impact directly over heart
- Precise timing of blow to a narrow 15 ms segment of the cardiac cycle vulnerable to potentially lethal ventricular arrhythmias just before the T wave peak
- Narrow, compliant chest wall, typical of young children.

> Most commotio cordis events are fatal; however, a few athletes survive, supporting the importance of early recognition and prompt institution of cardiopulmonary resuscitation and defibrillation[4]

Arrhythmias and athletes

Cardiac arrhythmias in athletes range from the benign and asymptomatic to symptomatic and potentially life threatening. Supraventricular and ventricular extrasystoles are common and usually are of no clinical significance. The high vagal tone associated with physical training may result in athletes being more susceptible to certain bradyarrhythmias. Asymptomatic bradyarrhythmias such as sinus bradycardia, nodal bradycardia, and second degree atrioventricular block (Mobitz I) are common among athletes and are caused by the high vagal tone associated with intense physical training. Higher degrees of atrioventricular block are very uncommon and treatable by pacing. Supraventricular arrhythmias are uncommon in athletes and should be treated with electrophysiological radiofrequency ablation. In a small number of athletes, high vagal tone may predispose to atrial fibrillation.[6]

Potentially life threatening ventricular arrhythmias are uncommon in athletes and generally are associated with underlying structural heart disease, coronary artery disease, or ion channelopathies. In these circumstances, participation in sport of high and moderate intensities is contraindicated. In a few cases, ventricular tachycardia may occur in the absence of these predisposing substrates, when it is amenable to treatment with electrophysiological radiofrequency ablation.

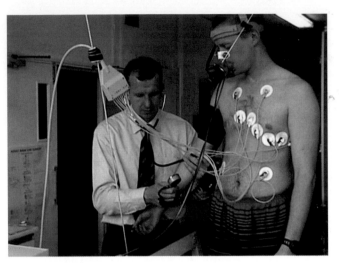

Integrated cardiopulmonary stress test in an athlete

Pathological cardiac causes of exertional syncope

- Ventricular tachycardia
- Ventricular obstruction resulting from aortic stenosis or hypertrophic cardiomyopathy
- Hypotension caused by vagally mediated vasodepression in patients with hypertrophic cardiomyopathy

Syncope and athletes

Unexplained syncope in an athlete is a potentially ominous symptom that needs thorough cardiovascular evaluation. The most frequent cause is neurocardiogenic (vasovagal); syncope is usually caused by neurally mediated mechanisms but may be compounded by dehydration. Most cases occur in the absence of an underlying cardiac cause; however, structural heart disease and other causes should be eliminated before considering neurocardiogenic syncope as the aetiology. Exercise testing is useful and should be performed while recording electrocardiograms during the sport in which the athlete participates. Athletes with syncope associated with exercise who have a fully negative cardiac evaluation can safely participate in sport of all types and intensities. The exception to this rule is any person with recurrent syncope who participates in sports where even transient loss of consciousness may be hazardous.

Traditional pharmacotherapy for vasovagal syndrome includes β_1 adrenergic blocking agents, antiarrhythmics, and plasma volume expanders. These groups of drugs currently are prohibited by international governing bodies of sport. In addition, care must be taken when prescribing drugs that possess negative inotropic actions. Strategies to reduce or eliminate vasovagal symptoms are targeted at maintaining blood pressure and venous return after exercise, including warm down, coughing, muscle tensing, and leg crossing.[8]

> Syncope in an athlete should always be followed up by a full cardiovascular work up. Postexercise syncope is more prevalent in endurance trained athletes and, in the presence of a negative cardiovascular work up, is benign
>
> Where the athlete is in danger of impact injury or drowning, however, treatment strategies are crucial. When pharmacotherapy is unnecessary or restricted, continuation of exercise and lower body positive pressure manoeuvres after exercise limits or eliminates the prevalence of syncope

Emergency medical care and athlete evaluation

Sudden cardiac death in sport is preventable. Unfortunately, most athletes who collapse during or immediately after sport die because cardiopulmonary resuscitation often is delayed. Facilities to deal with cardiac events should be available at training and competition venues. These facilities should include personnel trained in advanced life support and the provision of external automated cardiovertor defibrillators. Personnel responsible for athletes during training and competition should also receive training in basic and advanced life support.

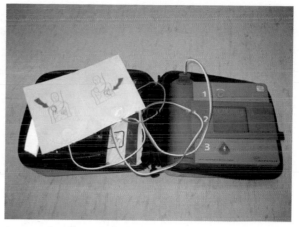

Automated cardiovertor defibrillators should be available at all training and competition venues

1 Sharma S, Whyte G, Elliott PM, Padula M, Kaushal R, Mahon N, et al. Electrocardiographic changes in 1000 highly trained elite athletes. *Br J Sports Med* 1999;30:319-24

2 Pelliccia A, Maron BJ, Spataro A, Proschan M, Spirito P. The upper limits of physiologic cardiac hypertrophy in highly trained athletes. *N Engl J Med* 1991;324:295-301

3 Whyte G, George K, Sharma S, Firoozi S, Stephens N, Senior R, et al. The upper limit of physiologic cardiac hypertrophy in elite male and female athletes: the British experience. *Eur J Appl Physiol* 2004;31:592-7

4 Maron BJ. The young competitive athlete with cardiovascular abnormalities: causes of sudden death, detection by preparticipation screening, and standards for disqualification. *Cardiac Electrophys Rev* 2002;6:100-3

5 Sharma S, Elliott PM, Whyte G, Mahon N, McKenna WJ. Physiologic limits of left ventricular hypertrophy in elite junior athletes: relevance to differential diagnosis of athlete's heart and hypertrophic cardiomyopathy. *J Am Coll Cardiol* 2002;40:1431-6

6 Whyte G, Stephens N, Budgett R, Sharma S, Shave R, McKenna W. Spontaneous atrial fibrillation in a freestyle skier. *Br J Sports Med* 2004;38:230-2

7 Corrado D, Basso C, Schiavon M, Thiene G. Screening for hypertrophic cardiomyopathy in young athletes. *N Engl J Med* 1998;339:364-9

8 Krediet P, van Dijk N, Linzer M, van Lieshout J, Wieling W. Management of vasovagal syncope: controlling or aborting faints by leg crossing and muscle tensing. *Circulation* 2002;106:1684-9

Further reading

- Link M, Homoud M, Wang P, Estes M. Cardiac arrhythmias in the athlete. *Cardiol Rev* 2001;9:21-30
- Maron BJ, Shirani J, Poliac LC, Mathenge R, Roberts WC, Mueller FO. Sudden death in young competitive athletes. Clinical, demographic and pathological profiles. *JAMA* 1996;276:199-204

13   Environmental factors

Mike Tipton

Since the 5th century BC when Herodicus was advocating good diet for physical training, the influence of nutrition on sporting performance has been a predominant and enduring theme. In contrast, the influence of the environment on sporting performance is a relatively recent consideration, and one that often is overlooked. Yet, environmental influences can have an enormous impact on performance and safety. This chapter reviews the influences of heat, cold, and altitude on the body.

Temperature

Thermal balance

Heat is exchanged between the body and the environment by four physical processes: convection (C), conduction (K), radiation (R), and evaporation (E). To remain in thermal balance, the heat gained by the body must equal that lost, such that no heat is stored (S) in the body.

The catabolic chemical reactions of the body liberate energy; the sum total of which constitutes total metabolic energy utilisation or rate (M). The biggest cause of variation in energy expenditure comes with muscle activity, such as exercise or shivering. Only 20-25% of the chemical energy used during muscular contraction is converted into mechanical work—the remainder is liberated as heat; during sustained vigorous exercise, heat production can reach in excess of 20 kcal.min^{-1}.

The thermoregulatory system of the body is a complex mix of cold and warm receptors, afferent and efferent pathways, central nervous system integrating and controlling centres, and effectors. The primary aim of this system is to maintain body temperature within safe limits. In air at 25-28°C, or water at 35°C, a naked, resting person can maintain body temperature by varying the amount of heat delivered to the skin through the circulation; in this situation, cutaneous blood flow averages 250 ml.min^{-1}. As air or water temperature falls or increases, shivering or sweating is initiated in an attempt to defend body temperature. These autonomic responses are costly in terms of substrate and fluid and only have a limited capability to defend body temperature when compared with behaviour.

Heat

Human skin contains 2-4 million sweat glands—more per unit area than any other mammal. These sweat glands are activated within seconds of exercise starting and reach maximum output after about 30 minutes. Sweat is a hypotonic saline solution containing 0.3-0.6% sodium chloride. In a hot environment (above body temperature), heat produced by metabolism and that gained by conduction, convection, and radiation must be matched by that lost by evaporation. This emphasises the importance of the evaporation of sweat in a hot environment.

For the deep body temperature of a person to increase to a new steady state level during exercise in air is normal. This is thought to be a regulated rise that is similar in magnitude between people when they work at the same relative work load (% VO$_{2max}$) and represents an adjustment that optimises metabolic function. The body temperature attained during exercise is dependent on work rate (up to 65% VO$_{2max}$) but independent of ambient conditions over a range of temperatures (5-25°C) with relatively low humidity ("prescriptive zone"). Above the prescriptive zone, deep body temperature rises.

Over the past 20 years, numerous climbers have died from acute mountain sickness, cold water immersion remains the largest killer of sports people engaged in their sport, and more than 100 American footballers have died from excessive heat stress

Heat balance equation

$$M - (W) = R \pm C \pm K - E$$

M = metabolic energy utilisation (metabolic rate)
W is measurable external work

The unit for each term is W.m^{-2}

If the body was prevented from losing any of the heat it produced during exercise, a fatal level of heat storage would be reached in about four hours when at rest and after just 25 minutes with moderate exercise

Whenever possible in air, body temperature is kept within about 1°C of 37°C and skin temperature averages 33°C. Humans can survive a fall in core temperature of around 10°C (this figure can vary dramatically) and an increase of about 6°C

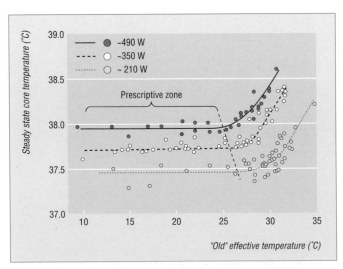

The prescriptive zone—effective temperature is the temperature of still, unsaturated air that gives rise to a thermal sensation that is equivalent to that evoked in other environments with different temperatures and different humidities. Adapted from Lind AR. *J Appl Physiol* 1963;18:51-6

Effects on performance

Exercise in the heat places an additional strain on the cardiovascular system. Heat dissipation during moderate to severe exercise in the heat occurs more by repartitioning cardiac output rather than by increasing it: 15-25% of cardiac output is directed to the skin to assist in heat loss and constriction of splanchnic and renal vascular beds enables most of this increase in cutaneous blood flow.

Heart rate is unable to offset the fall in stroke volume during maximal exercise in the heat; as a consequence, maximal cardiac output falls. This limits the ability of unacclimatised people to exercise in such conditions. The VO_{2max} usually is reported to be lower in hot climates than temperate climates.

Submaximal exercise performance can also be affected: marathon performance declines by about 1 minute for each 1°C increase in air temperature above 15°C. Compromised muscle blood flow and decreased hepatic blood flow result in an earlier onset of anaerobic metabolism and blood lactate accumulation. Use of glycogen in muscle is increased and fatigue occurs earlier during prolonged moderate exercise in the heat. A diminished central drive to exercise is seen in hyperthermic people. Heat does not decrease maximum strength, but it does reduce muscle endurance and time to fatigue.

Aerobically fit people are able to perform for longer in hot environments and tolerate higher levels of hyperthermia than less fit people. Abnormally high core temperatures, however, impair exercise performance in all people in the heat.

Dehydration during exercise in the heat

During exercise, body fluid loss, primarily caused by sweating, increases by an amount that depends on several factors. An athlete training in a hot climate may need to drink 4-12 litres a day.

In comparison with the responses seen when hydrated, fluid loss equivalent to 1% of body mass increases rectal temperature. Dehydration equivalent to 5% of body mass increases rectal temperature because of decreased sweating and cutaneous blood flow. Dehydration between 1.9-4.3% of body mass can reduce endurance by 22-48% and VO_{2max} by 10-22%.

The risk of heat illness is increased if exercise is undertaken in the heat in a dehydrated state.

Heat illness

The problems caused by heat result from:

- Decreased circulating blood volume and consequent alterations in regional blood flow
- Increased blood viscosity
- Direct effect of temperature on respiratory centres and proteins

Heat illness can occur in cool or temperate conditions if humidity is high or if people are unable to offload the heat produced from high work rates because of clothing. A large list of factors influences thermoregulation and a person's susceptibility to heat illness. Some of these can operate acutely (for example, infection), so a person may have heat illness in circumstances in which they were previously unaffected.

Strategies to maintain performance and avoid heat illness
Maintaining fluid balance
The signs of dehydration, which include fatigue, headache, irritability, and insomnia are important to recognise. Clearly, a person is disadvantaged if they begin exercise in the heat in a dehydrated state. To "adapt" to low water intake is not possible and should not be attempted.

Cardiovascular responses of unacclimatised men walking for 15 minutes at 10% gradient in 26°C and 43°C

Response at 43°C compared with 26°C
- Central blood volume—16% lower
- Oxygen consumption—same
- Heart rate—15% higher
- a-vO$_2$ difference—no substantial difference
- Stroke volume—same

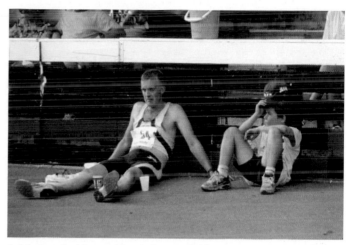

A dehydrated athlete—without adequate fluid replacement, sportsmen can lose an amount of body fluid equivalent to 3-10% of their body mass while exercising

---

Factors that determine body fluid loss during exercise

- Environmental temperature
- Fitness
- Level of acclimatisation
- Intensity of activity
- Duration of the activity

Factors that influence thermoregulation and susceptibility to heat illness

- Air temperature, humidity, movement, and radiant heat load
- Body size (mass and skinfold thickness)—heat stroke occurs 3.5 times more often in excessively overweight young adults than in people of average body mass
- State of training or sudden increase in training (military recruits with low aerobic fitness (>12 minutes for a 1.5 mile run) and a high body mass index (>26) have a ninefold greater risk of heat illness)
- Degree of acclimatisation
- Hydration status
- Heat production (exercise intensity or duration)
- Clothing worn (vapour permeability, fit, and colour)
- State of health (for example, fever, viral illness, cold, flu, diabetes mellitus, cardiovascular disease, gastroenteritis, and diarrhoea)
- Genetic disorders (for example, mutations for cystic fibrosis and malignant hyperthermia)
- Skin disorders, for example, sunburn on more than 5% of body surface area
- Use of drugs (such as diuretics; antihistamines; ergogenic stimulants)
- Sweat gland dysfunction (for example, prickly heat)
- Salt depletion
- Age
- Sleep deprivation
- Glycogen or glucose depletion
- Acute or chronic alcohol or drug abuse

Heat illness

Heat exhaustion
- Most common form of heat illness, defined as inability to continue exercise in heat
- Usually seen in unacclimatised people
- Caused by ineffective circulatory adjustments and reduced blood volume
- Characterised by: breathlessness, hyperventilation, weak and rapid pulse, low blood pressure, dizziness, headache, flushed skin, nausea, paradoxical chills, irritability, lethargy, general weakness
- Deep body temperature is raised but not excessively, sweating persists, and no organ damage occurs
- People with heat exhaustion should: stop exercising, lie down, control breathing if hyperventilating, rehydrate
- Failure to do so can result in progression to severe heat illness
- Heat exhaustion is a predominant problem when body water loss exceeds 7% of body mass

Heat stroke
- Medical emergency resulting from failure of the thermoregulatory system as a result of a high deep body temperature (>40.5°C)
- Characterised by: confusion, absence of sweating, hot and dry skin, circulatory instability
- If not treated by immediate cooling, results in death from circulatory collapse and multiorgan damage
- Aggressive steps should be taken to cool the casualty, as mortality is related to the degree and duration of hyperthermia:
  Consider using "artificial sweat" (spraying with tepid water or alcohol) and fanning and fluid replacement (do not overinfuse or overload, as this can result in pulmonary oedema)
  Consider colder water immersion/ice packs for those without a peripheral circulation
- Heat stroke should be the working diagnosis in anyone who has an altered mental state
- Deep body temperature should be monitored every five minutes; deep (15 cm) rectal temperature is preferable to mouth or ear canal as these may be influenced by hyperventilation or the active cooling strategy employed, or both
- People with heat exhaustion should improve rapidly with appropriate immediate care; any who do not improve quickly should be evacuated to the next level of medical care
- Recovery from exertional heat stroke is idiosyncratic and in severe cases may take up to a year

Heat cramps
- Usually occur in the specific muscles exercised because of an imbalance in the body's fluid volume and electrolyte concentration and low energy stores
- Core temperature remains in normal range
- Aetiology unknown
- Can be prevented by an appropriate rehydration strategy
- Treated by stretching and massage

Exertional rhabdomyolysis
- Caused by muscle damage resulting in the release of cellular contents (for example, myoglobin, potassium, phosphate, creatine kinase and uric acid) into the circulation
- More likely if dehydrated or taking non-steroidal anti-inflammatory drugs
- Overt signs include muscle pain, tenderness, weakness, and very dark urine
- Treat by giving fluids, evacuate to intensive medical care, kidney function should be assessed

General principles of fluid replacement
- Sweat is hypotonic in comparison with body fluids, so water rather than mineral replacement is the primary concern
- Water absorption occurs mainly in the upper part of the small intestine and depends on osmotic gradients:
  Addition of small amounts of glucose and sodium to a rehydration drink has little negative effect on gastric emptying
  Presence of glucose may accelerate fluid uptake because of the active cotransport of glucose and sodium across the intestinal mucosa
  Addition of sodium will help to maintain plasma sodium concentrations, reduce urine output, and sustain the sodium dependent osmotic drive to drink
- Drinks with low sugar content (2-4% (20-40 g/l)) will not supply much energy, but if they are hypotonic and have a high sodium content (40-60 mmol/l (1-1.5 g/l)), they will give the fastest water replacement. The fastest rate of energy supply is achieved with high sugar concentrations (15-20% (150-200 g/l)), but this limits the rate at which water is absorbed
- Gastric emptying slows when ingested fluids have high osmolality (plasma osmolality = 280 mOsm/l) or caloric content. A drink that contains glucose polymers rather than simple sugars minimises this negative effect
- Gastric volume influences gastric emptying, with the rate of emptying increasing with volume in the stomach. Consumption of 400-600 ml immediately before exercise optimises the transfer of fluids into the intestine. Drinking 150-250 ml at 15 minute intervals during exercise maintains gastric volume and fluid uptake at maximal levels of about 1 litre per hour
- A drink that tastes good is more likely to be drunk
- Highly carbonated beverages retard gastric emptying

Overhydration and hyponatraemia
- Athletes should not drink as much as they can in the belief that more is better. Concerns about excessive overhydration and hyponatraemia (low blood sodium) among endurance athletes has led the American track and field governing body to urge runners to hydrate based on individual need. One post-race study of 481 runners in the 2002 Boston Marathon suggested that 13% experienced hyponatraemia; one woman died from hyponatraemic encephalopathy. This is somewhat higher than the 0.31% reported after the Houston Marathon in 2000. Nevertheless, hyponatraemia is a condition that, according to the medical literature, has been responsible for at least seven deaths and 250 cases
- Risk factors include:
  Being a woman with slow finishing times in long duration events (running speed < 5 mph)
  Excessive fluid consumption (15 l in 5-6 hours of exercise)
  Underreplacement of sodium loss
- Hyponatraemia can result in intracellular swelling that, if severe enough, can produce symptoms of central nervous dysfunction, lung congestion, and muscle weakness
- Hyponatraemia and dehydration mediated heat exhaustion share many symptoms and laboratory tests are needed to distinguish between the two. Patients with dehydration mediated heat exhaustion respond fairly quickly to fluid replacement, whereas the condition of those with hyponatraemia will be aggravated by hypotonic fluids
- The International Marathon Medical Directors Association (IMMDA, 2002) stated that blanket hydration recommendations for athletes are incorrect and unsafe and that athletes should drink as needed but not exceed 400-800 ml per hour, with lesser amounts drunk for slower, smaller athletes in mild environments and greater amounts for faster athletes in warmer environments

The upper rate at which fluid will empty from the stomach during exercise is 1-1.5 litres per hour; even the most effective oral fluid replacement strategies will fail to prevent dehydration above this level of sweat loss. Volitionally, most people replace only about half of the fluid they need to rehydrate, as thirst is quenched at this level of rehydration.

Body cooling

The benefit of whole body precooling seems to be dependent on environment and activity. It is not beneficial in simulated triathlons or football related activities under normal environments. In contrast, precooling to reduce core temperature by 0.7°C (for example, immersion in cool (23°C) water) has been shown to increase subsequent exercise endurance in hot and humid conditions, with time to exhaustion being related inversely to initial body temperature. Cooling the skin by just 5-6°C reduces thermal strain and increases cycling performance (distance cycled in 30 minutes) in warm and humid conditions.

Returning body temperature to normal levels between repeated bouts of exercise in the heat helps to maintain performance, decreases physiological strain, and extends work time. One of the quickest and simplest ways of doing this is by hand immersion in cold water: the large surface area and high cutaneous blood flow of the hands make them ideal for heat exchange. The rates of heat exchange achieved by this method compare favourably with those achieved with the use of ice vests or forced convective cooling.

Acclimatisation

Repeated exposure to hot environments that produce increases in deep body and skin temperature and profuse sweating result in acclimatisation to heat, which improves exercise capacity and comfort. Exercise during these exposures (gradually increasing exercise intensity each day until at normal pace) is important, as resting in the heat provides only partial acclimatisation. The acclimatisation is specific to the climate and activity level; people acclimatised to hot dry environments will need additional time to acclimatise if they move to hot humid environments.

The process needs exposure to representative environmental temperatures for at least two hours a day, and takes a total of 10-14 days. No more than three days should elapse between successive exposures. The adjustments to the raised body temperatures associated with exercise mean that fitter individuals can acclimatise more quickly (7-10 days). Even fit people need to exercise in a hot environment, however, to achieve full acclimatisation. The exposures can be in the field (acclimatisation) or in a suitable climatic chamber (acclimation). Use of sweat suits (impermeable or semi-permeable clothing) or saunas is partially effective. An acclimatised person can produce more sweat, so they have a greater fluid requirement to maintain hydration.

Beneficial changes associated with heat acclimatisation

- Increased plasma volume
- Less cardiovascular strain
- More effective distribution of cardiac output
- Improved cutaneous blood flow
- Earlier onset and great rate of sweating
- Lowered salt content in sweat (for example, sodium in sweat reduced from 50 to 25 mmol/l)
- More effective distribution of sweat over the skin surface
- Lower skin and deep body temperatures for a given level of exercise
- Improved physical work capacity
- Increased comfort
- Decreased reliance on carbohydrate metabolism

Assessing the risk of a warm environment

- The most widely used heat stress index is the wet bulb globe temperature (WBGT) index. The formula for this is:
  $$WBGT = 0.1T_{db} + 0.7T_{wb} + 0.2T_g$$
  T_{db} = dry bulb temperature, T_{wb} = wet bulb temperature, and T_g = globe temperature
- The weightings emphasise the importance of humidity for heat stress
- Meters for measuring wet bulb globe temperature can be bought relatively inexpensively. They consist of:
  Thermometer or thermistor (dry bulb)
  Thermometer or thermistor covered with a dampened wick (wet bulb)
  Thermometer or thermistor enclosed on a black metal sphere that absorbs radiant energy from the surroundings (globe temperature)

Recommendations

- Recommendations to reduce the chance of heat injury in athletic activity in lightly clothed individuals:
  26.5-28.8°C—Use discretion, especially if untrained or unacclimatised
  29.5-30.5°C—Avoid strenuous activity in the sun
  >31.2°C—Avoid exercise training
- For sportspeople who wear heavier clothing, the lower temperature in each range should be used
- The American College of Sports Medicine recommendations for continuous activities such as running and cycling according to the wet bulb globe temperature are:
  <18°C—Low risk
  18-23°C—Moderate risk
  23-28°C—High risk: those with predisposing factors for heat illness should not compete
  >28°C—Very high risk: postpone competition
- The optimum temperature for prolonged strenuous exercise (cycle ergometry), as assessed by time to exhaustion, is 11°C. This time is reduced by 13% at 21°C and 45% at 31°C

On return to a temperate climate, the major benefits of heat acclimatisation are retained for a week. Within three weeks of returning, 75% of the benefits are lost

---

Clothing in heat

- To minimise thermal burden, clothing should be:
  Lightweight—to minimise insulation and increase exchange of air between microclimate (beneath clothing) and environment with body movement ("Bellows effect")
  Light coloured—to reflect more radiant heat
  Loose—to facilitate Bellows effect
  Vapour permeable—to facilitate evaporative heat loss
  Made from materials that readily absorb water (for example, linen or cotton)—to facilitate evaporative heat loss
- Protective clothing worn for sporting activities can impose a substantial thermal load on body and result in substantially higher skin and deep body temperatures. Combination of insulative clothing and high levels of metabolic heat production has resulted in cases of fatal heat stroke

Cold

Although air temperature can fall to lower levels than water temperature, water represents the greater threat because of its higher thermal conductivity and specific heat. In most circumstances in air, the heat produced by exercise is enough to offset that lost to a cold environment, particularly when combined with the careful use of clothing. In air therefore, problems with cooling tend to arise only when heat production is reduced because of injury or exhaustion. In contrast, exercise tends to accelerate rather than prevent cooling in cold water: the heat produced by exercise does not balance the increased heat lost because of moving in the water and increasing blood flow to the person's peripheral musculature.

Effects on performance
In air or water, the first tissue to be affected on exposure to cold is the skin. Skin cooling is accentuated by peripheral vasoconstriction initiated by the body to reduce heat loss. The extremities (hands and feet) are most affected because of their high surface area to mass ratio and because their major source of heat—blood flow—is restricted by vasoconstriction. This partly explains why the extremities normally receive cold injuries. Rapid skin cooling on immersion in cold water evokes a set of cardiorespiratory responses that can be precursors to cardiovascular accidents and drowning.

The next tissues to cool are the superficial nerves and muscles. This can result in physical incapacitation. The time taken for this to occur depends on the exact nature of the environment (air or water, temperature, and wind speed). The conduction of action potentials is slowed (15 m/s per 10°C fall in local temperature) and their amplitude reduced. Below a muscle temperature of 27°C, the contractile force and rate of force application is reduced, and fatigue occurs earlier—maximum power output falls by 3% per 1°C fall in muscle temperature. As a consequence, speed of movement, dexterity, strength, and mechanical efficiency all are reduced with cooling.

In cold water, a fall in deep body temperature intensifies shivering, which raises oxygen consumption during submaximal exercise (9% in water at 25°C and 25.3% in water at 18°C). The increase is greater in leaner people. The energy cost of submaximal exercise thus is higher in water cooler than 26°C; this can result in more rapid depletion of carbohydrate and lipid energy sources and earlier onset of fatigue.

When shivering occurs during exercise in the cold, cardiac output is elevated above levels seen during exercise in temperate conditions. Stroke volume usually is higher and heart rate lower during exercise in the cold because of increased central blood volume and cardiac preload as a result of peripheral vasoconstriction.

VO_{2max}, during ergometry or swimming and maximum performance are both reduced during cold water immersion. This reduction occurs in water with a temperature as high as 25°C and is roughly linearly related to deep body temperature, with a 10-30% reduction seen after a 0.5-2°C fall in deep body temperature. Associated with this reduction in VO_{2max}, lactate appears in the blood at lower workloads and accumulates at a more rapid rate than in thermoneutral conditions. This suggests that oxygen delivery to the working muscles is reduced during profound cooling. This situation may be accentuated by a left shift in the oxygen dissociation curve with cooling. A decrease in deep body temperature of 0.5-1.5°C results in a reduction of 10-40% in the capacity to supply oxygen to meet the increased needs of activity. With more profound cooling, anaerobic metabolism also is reduced because of muscle cooling and direct impairment of the processes responsible for the anaerobic production of energy.

> Skin temperature cools rapidly on immersion in cold water, and the deep body temperature of a person immersed in cold water will cool about four times faster than when in air of the same temperature

Some cardiorespiratory responses to rapid skin cooling in cold water
- Uncontrollable hyperventilation
- Hypertension
- Increased cardiac workload

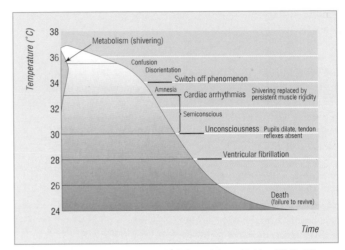

Signs and symptoms of hypothermia. Adapted from Golden FStC. *J Roy Naval Med* 1973;59:5-8

> The combination of exhaustion, hypoglycaemia, dehydration and hypothermia can represent a serious threat during exposure to the cold

Hypothermia
Hypothermia exists when deep body temperature falls below 35°C. Risk factors for hypothermia include:
- Cold air or water temperature
- Air or water movement: faster moving fluids increase convective heat loss
- Age: children cool faster than adults because of their lower levels of subcutaneous fat and higher surface area to mass ratio
- Body stature: tall, thin people cool faster than short, fat people
- Body morphology: body fat and unperfused muscle are good insulators
- Sex: females tend to have more subcutaneous fat than men
- Fitness: high fitness enables higher heat production
- Fatigue: exhaustion results in decreased heat production
- Nutritional state: hypoglycaemia attenuates shivering and accentuates cooling
- Intoxication: drug or alcohol depressant effects on metabolism
- Lack of appropriate clothing

Dehydration is common in cold environments because thirst is blunted, water is not always easily available (frozen), and respiratory water loss can be high in cold dry environments. Furthermore, cold exposure can result in a cold induced diuresis because of raised central venous pressure; this is prevented by moderate exercise in the cold.

Acclimatisation to cold

A good deal of debate still exists about whether humans can acclimatise to cold. Various forms of adaptation have been described in the literature, none of which seems particularly beneficial. The most frequently reported adaptation to cold is characterised by a reduced shivering response (habituation), faster fall in deep body temperature (hypothermic adaptation), and increased thermal comfort. This is typically seen in outdoor long distance swimmers.

The hazardous initial responses to immersion in cold water can be reduced by as much as 50% by as few as five two minute immersions in cold water. A large part of this habituation seems to last for months.

Cold injury

Cold injuries can be of the "freezing" (frostbite) or non-freezing variety (non-freezing cold injury).

Human tissue freezes at around −0.55°C and depending on the rate of freezing, intracellular crystals may form (rapid cooling) causing direct mechanical disruption of the tissues. Slow cooling and freezing is more common and results in predominantly extracellular water crystallisation that increases plasma and interstitial fluid osmotic pressure. The resulting osmotic outflow of intracellular fluid raises intracellular osmotic pressure and can cause damage to capillary walls. This, along with the local reduction in plasma volume, causes oedema and reduced local blood flow and encourages capillary sludging. These changes can produce thrombosis and gangrenous extremities.

Non-freezing cold injury is the term given to describe a condition that results from protracted exposure to low ambient thermal conditions but in which freezing of tissues does not occur.

The precise pathophysiology of non-freezing cold injury is poorly understood; the injury seems to be to the neuroendotheliomuscular components of the walls of local blood vessels. Opinions vary as to whether the primary damage is vascular or neural in origin or whether the aetiology is primarily thermal, ischaemic, post-ischaemic reperfusion, or hypoxic in origin. The chronic sequelae of mild to moderate cold injury are "cold sensitivity" (protracted cold vasoconstriction following a cold stimulus) and hyperhidrosis (local increased sweating), both of which accentuate local cooling and thus increase future risk of cold injury.

Treatment

To establish whether the dominant injury is freezing or non-freezing in nature is important, as this determines the preferred method of rewarming. In all cases, shelter should be sought. Because casualties with cold injury are likely to be hypothermic they should be kept warm.

All cases of freezing injury should be thoroughly rewarmed by immersion of all the chilled parts in stirred water at 38-42°C. A topical antibacterial also should be diluted into the water bath. Rewarming should be delayed if refreezing may occur. Thawing a freezing cold injury can be intensely painful. Conventional and narcotic analgesics should be provided as necessary. Continuing treatment for freezing cold injury

Clothing in cold

Clothing in the cold should:

- Prevent flushing of cold air or water beneath the garment—that is, have airtight or watertight seals
- Provide insulation by trapping a large volume of dry air close to the skin
- Enable adjustments in insulation to cater for times of increased and decreased metabolic heat production
- Be windproof
- Wick moisture away from the body for comfort
- Be vapour permeable to prevent accumulation and condensation of moisture under the clothing, which, because of its high thermal capacity, will reduce clothing insulation

When exercising in the cold, several layers of lighter clothing generally are considered to be better than one large bulky garment. The former approach enables clothing insulation to be adjusted more easily

Out of hospital treatment of hypothermia

- Lay casualty flat, give essential first aid, and enquire about coexisting illness
- Prevent further heat loss (blankets or sleeping bag), cover head, and leave airway clear
- Insulate from the ground
- If possible, provide shelter from the wind and rain
- Allow slow spontaneous rewarming to occur: rewarming too quickly can result in rewarming collapse
- Maintain close observation of pulse and respiration
- Obtain help as soon as possible and transport the casualty to hospital
- If breathing is absent, becomes obstructed, or stops, standard expired air ventilation should be instituted
- Chest compression should only be started if:
  — no carotid pulse is detectable after palpating for at least one minute (pulse is slow and weak in hypothermia), and
  — cardiac arrest is observed or may reasonably have occurred within the previous two hours, and
  — effective cardiopulmonary resuscitation can reasonably be expected to be provided continuously until the casualty reaches more advanced life support; this is likely to mean being within two hours of a suitable hospital
- The rates of expired air ventilation and chest compression should be the same as for normothermic casualties. Hypothermia may cause stiffness of the chest wall

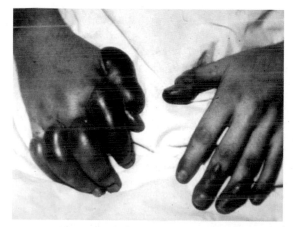

Frostbite—risk of frostbite is low at air temperatures higher than −7°C, irrespective of wind speed, and becomes pronounced when ambient temperature is lower than −25°C, even at low wind speeds

comprises twice daily, 30 minute immersion of the affected part in a whirlpool bath containing an appropriate antibacterial at 38-42°C.

In contrast to those with freezing cold injury, the affected extremities of patients with non-freezing cold injury should be rewarmed slowly by exposure to warm air alone and must not be immersed in warm water. The early period after rewarming can be very painful for patients with non-freezing cold injury, even in those without any obvious tissue damage. Amitriptyline (10-75 mg in a single dose at night) is the drug of choice for the treatment of pain after non-freezing cold injury and should be given as soon as pain is felt. Amitriptyline may cause drowsiness and hypertension.

With either form of injury, once rewarmed, the affected extremities should be treated by exposure to air and early mobilisation. Smoking should be prohibited.

Assessing the risk of cold injuries

The cooling power of the environment is the result of air temperature and air movement or movement through air (for example, when skiing). These factors are combined into the wind chill index, which illustrates the cooling effect of temperature and wind on bare skin and predicts the associated danger of cold injury.

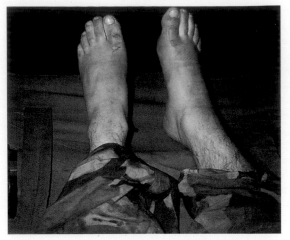

Non-freezing cold injury—immobility, posture, dehydration, low fitness, inadequate nutrition, constricting footwear, fatigue, stress or anxiety, and concurrent illness or injury all can increase the likelihood of non-freezing cold injury

Altitude

The low air temperatures at altitude increase the likelihood of cold related injuries and result in low absolute humidity. Air temperature falls by about 1°C with every 150 m (490 ft) of ascent. This predisposes to dehydration, as a large volume of body water can be lost through the respiratory tract as dry cold air is warmed and humidified with body water during breathing. Although temperature falls with altitude, solar radiation increases, because there is less atmosphere and water to absorb the radiation.

Barometric pressure at a given point is related to the weight of air in the atmosphere above that point. The relation between altitude and barometric pressure is exponential rather than linear because air is compressible. One atmosphere is the pressure exerted by about 24 miles (38.6 km) of air above us and is equal to about 760 mm Hg (101.325 kPa, 14.696 psi).

Longer term adjustments to altitude

- Hyperventilation
- Excretion of excess base (HCO_3^-) via the kidneys—reduced alkaline reserve
- Submaximal heart rate remains elevated
- Submaximal cardiac output falls lower than sea level values
- Stroke volume decreases
- Maximum cardiac output decreases
- VO_{2max} reduced less
- Arteriovenous oxygen difference (a-vO_2) increases
- Decreased plasma volume, which is then restored
- Increased haematocrit
- Increased haemoglobin concentration
- Increased total number of red blood cells
- Increased 2,3-diphosphoglycerate in red blood cells
- Increased mitochondrial density
- Increased aerobic enzymes in muscle
- Loss of lean body mass and body mass
- Excretion rates and plasma level of norepinephrine increase (increased sympathoadrenal activity)
- Appetite and weight loss
- Increased capillaries per unit volume

Wind chill chart: effect of increasing wind speed on degree of cooling at different ambient temperatures

Wind speed (mph)	Ambient temperature (°C)									
	4	−1	−7	−12	−18	−23	−29	−34	−40	−46
	*Wind chill (equivalent) temperature (°C)**									
5	2	−4	−12	−15	−21	−26	−32	−37	−43	−48
10	−1	−9	−15	−23	−29	−37	−34	−51	−57	−62
15	−4	−12	−21	−29	−34	−43	−51	−57	−65	−73
20	−7	−15	−23	−32	−37	−46	−54	−62	−71	−79
25	−9	−18	−26	−34	−43	−51	−59	−68	−76	−84
30	−12	−18	−29	−34	−46	−54	−62	−71	−79	−87
35	−12	−21	−29	−37	−46	−54	−62	−73	−82	−90
40	−12	−21	−29	−37	−48	−57	−65	−73	−82	−90

Less danger	Increasing danger. Flesh may freeze within a minute	Great danger. Flesh may freeze within 30 seconds

*Equivalent temperature is the environmental temperature that would have the same effect on bare skin in the absence of any wind (equivalent cooling power)

Immediate adjustments to altitude

- Hyperventilation and respiratory alkalosis
- Body fluids become more alkaline
- Increase in submaximal heart rate
- Increase in submaximal cardiac output
- Stroke volume the same or slight decrease
- Maximum cardiac output, stroke volume, and heart rate reduced
- VO_{2max} reduced
- Higher lactic acid production for given submaximal work rates
- Lower lactic acid production at maximal work rates

The fractional concentrations of the gases in air remain unchanged with increasing altitude (20.93% oxygen, 79.04% nitrogen, and 0.03% carbon dioxide), but the partial pressures of the gases in air fall in direct proportion to the fall in barometric pressure. The reduction in partial pressure of oxygen (density of oxygen molecules) with increasing altitude causes the decrements in performance by reducing oxygen transport in the tissues.

Effects on performance

Few physiological effects on performance are observed in unacclimatised people below an altitude of 1500 m. Influence of altitude on performance will then depend on the event:

- Sprinting and throwing events improve because of decreased air density and resistance (24% reduction in air density at 2300 m)
- Anaerobic events are unaffected
- Aerobic events are impaired by decreased aerobic capacity and increased fatigue.

Above 1600 m, VO_{2max} decreases by about 11% for every 1000 m increase in altitude up to 6300 m, when it starts to decline at a more rapid non-linear rate. For work at the same percentage of VO_{2max}, a 10% reduction in endurance run time has been reported on the first day after arrival at 4300 m.

High altitude pulmonary oedema

- High altitude pulmonary oedema occurs in about 2% of people who travel above 3000 m. The accumulation of fluid in the lungs is life threatening, causing breathlessness and fatigue, a dry and then productive cough with white sputum tinged with blood, chest discomfort, crackles at the lung bases, increased heart and respiratory rates, peripheral oedema, cyanosis, mental confusion, coma, and death in a few hours if untreated
- The cause is unknown, but high altitude pulmonary oedema seems to occur most frequently in those who rapidly ascend to altitudes above 2700 m and in children and young adults. A brisk pulmonary artery pressor response to hypoxia may be a risk factor
- High altitude pulmonary oedema is treated by supplemental oxygen and immediate evacuation to a lower altitude (at least 1000 m lower). A portable, lightweight, rubberised canvas hyperbaric chamber (Gamow bag) is available; this is pressurised to 2 psi with a foot pump and is equivalent to reducing altitude by 2000 m if at 4000-4500 m
- Nifedipine—a calcium channel blocker that decreases blood pressure (vasodilator)—can be beneficial and should be given under medical supervision. A 20 mg slow release oral preparation every six hours is the recommended dose

Acclimatisation

With time, the body gradually but never completely adapts to the lower partial pressure of oxygen at altitude. The decrement seen in endurance performance and VO_{2max} can be reduced by acclimatisation: one study reported a 10% increase in VO_{2max} between day 1 and 14 at 4300 m. However, even people who have lived and trained at altitude for years never attain the VO_{2max} or level of performance they might achieve at sea level.

Athletes who must go from sea level to compete at altitude have two options. The first is to compete within 24 hours of arriving, before all of the detrimental physiological responses to altitude (dehydration, sleep loss) develop. This option is far from ideal. The alternative is to train at altitude before the event. Complete acclimatisation needs 4-6 weeks at 1500-3000 m; partial acclimatisation can be achieved in two weeks to altitudes up to 2300 m. Thereafter, each 610 m increase in altitude needs another week for acclimatisation up to 4600 m. Acclimatisation to one altitude provides only partial adaptation to higher altitudes. To increase aerobic capacity at sea level before going

Acute mountain sickness

- Characterised by headache, nausea, vomiting, malaise, dyspnoea, rapid pulse rate, and insomnia
- Incidence varies with altitude, rate of ascent and individual susceptibility (no way of predicting). Between 2500 m and 3000 m acute mountain sickness occurs in about 6.5% of men and 22.2% of women, with varying severity and symptoms. These percentages rise as altitude increases and have been reported to reach about 50% in people travelling to 4205-5500 m. Physical conditioning does not seem to provide any protection. Respiratory infection can predispose to acute mountain sickness
- Symptoms begin 3-96 hours after arrival at high altitude and can be incapacitating for several days. The simple or benign form lasts 3-5 days and will not reappear at the same altitude
- Cause is not understood fully; hypoxaemia and alkalosis have been implicated, and cerebral oedema is probably involved. People with a low ventilatory response to hypoxia may be most at risk: the consequent accumulation of carbon dioxide in the tissues might be responsible for some of the symptoms of acute mountain sickness
- Can be avoided by slowing the rate of ascent to altitude (no more than 300 m/day when above 3000 m) and resting at lower altitudes (1-2 days rest for each 600 m above 2400 m). A person should return to lower altitudes where possible at the first signs of acute mountain sickness. Those travelling above 3000 m should carry several days' supply of oxygen
- Acetazolamide (Diamox) reduces the symptoms of acute mountain sickness. It is a carbonic acid anhydrase inhibitor that acts as a respiratory stimulator. The recommended dose is 250 mg a day. People who know they are susceptible to acute mountain sickness should start the drug not less than 24 hours before a major gain in altitude is expected. Side effects include mild diuresis and paraesthesia of the fingers and toes. Drug use is not a substitute for proper acclimatisation

High altitude cerebral oedema

- High altitude cerebral oedema, which is indistinguishable from acute mountain sickness in the early stages, becomes likely when ataxia appears as a symptom
- Incidence is lower than for high altitude pulmonary oedema (1% of those above 2700 m). Most cases have been reported at altitudes greater than 4300 m (14 106 ft)
- It is caused by fluid accumulating in the cranial cavity, which results in mental confusion, pulmonary oedema, coma, and death in a few hours if untreated
- It is treated by supplemental oxygen and immediate evacuation to a lower altitude. Dexamethasone (Decadron), a synthetic adrenocorticoid with powerful anti-inflammatory properties, given intramuscularly at a dose of 4 mg in severe cases and orally in less severe cases helps to reduce cerebral oedema

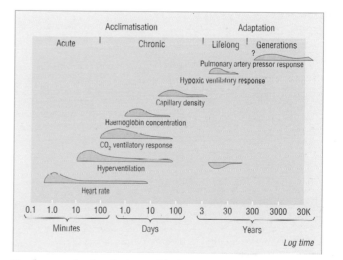

Time course of acclimatisation to altitude. Adapted from JS Milledge. Altitude. In: *Oxford textbook of medicine.* Oxford: Oxford University Press, 1998

to altitude can assist performance, as can starting full training as soon as possible at altitude; however, exercise intensity normally will need to be reduced during the first days at altitude and then increased over the first two weeks. Acclimatisation disappears within 2-3 weeks of returning to sea level.

Although a good theoretical argument supports the benefits of training at altitude before competition at sea level, most studies of highly trained individuals found no improvement in sea level performance after training at altitude; some improvements have been observed in less fit individuals. The difficulty of training at the same intensity at altitude, plus dehydration and weight loss, can all result in some detraining at altitude. This has led to the concept of train low and live high. By use of a hypoxic chamber, athletes can live at a preset altitude and obtain all of the beneficial adaptations to altitude but train at sea level to maintain the volume and intensity of their training programme. Such "live in" hypoxic chambers are becoming more common. It seems that longer than 1-2 hours a day must be spent breathing a hypoxic gas mixture if any adaptation is to be achieved.

We thank Dr A Allsopp, Dr FStC Golden, and Dr EHN Oakley. Photographs of frostbite and non-freezing cold injury are reproduced courtesy of the Cold Injuries Clinic, Institute of Naval Medicine, United Kingdom.

Further reading

- Francis TJR, Golden FStC. Non-freezing cold injury: the pathogenesis. *J Roy Naval Med Service* 1985;71:3-8
- Francis TJR, Oakley EHN. Cold injury. In: Tooke JE, Lowe GDO, eds. *A textbook of vascular medicine.* London: Arnold, 1996;353-70
- Golden FStC, Tipton MJ. *Essentials of sea survival.* Leeds: Human Kinetics, 2002
- Golden FStC. Death after rescue from immersion in cold water. *J Roy Naval Med Service* 1973;59:5-8
- Lind AR. A physiological criterion for setting thermal environmental limits for everyday work. *J Appl Physiol* 1963;18:51-6
- Milledge JS. Altitude. In: Harries M, Williams C, Stanish WD, Micheli LJ, eds. *Oxford textbook of sports medicine.* Oxford: Oxford University Press, 1998
- Oakley EHN. *A review of the treatment of cold injury. Institute of Naval Medicine report no. 2000.026.* Gosport: Institute of Naval Medicine, 2000
- Rowell LB, Marx HJ, Bruce RA, Conn RD, Kusumi F. Reductions in cardiac output, central blood volume, and stroke volume with thermal stress in normal men during exercise. *J Clin Invest* 1966;45:1801-16

14 Sports performance in a polluted environment

Geraint Florida-James, K Donaldson, Vicki Stone

Performing in a polluted environment

Exposures to raised levels of air pollution are associated widely with episodes of worsening lung disease and also deaths through impacts on the respiratory and cardiovascular systems. These "acute" effects are best documented within a few hours to a few days after the worsening of pollution in the climate. They are not seen uniformly throughout the population but instead are concentrated within susceptible subgroups with pre-existing disease. A "chronic" effect of air pollution also exists, however, and living in a polluted area increases the likelihood of developing airways disease, cardiovascular disease, and cancer compared with living in a less polluted area.

The impact of air pollution on athletic performance is likely to be important because of high ventilation rates that result in increased delivery of pollutants to the lungs, as well as subtle effects on physiology that result in serious effects on performance. Add to this the unique physiology of many elite athletes and the possibilities of an enhanced response to pollution exposure are amplified. A number of upcoming major competitions will take place in relatively polluted environments, so interest in the effects of pollution on athletic performance has increased.

Changing polluted environment

The adverse health effects of air pollution have been recognised for centuries. For example, in the ninth century, the burning of "sea coales" was recognised to generate intolerable noxious fumes in the city of London. In the thirteenth century, Edward I even banned the use of such fuels in London to prevent the accumulation of acrid smoke. In more recent times, burning of fossil fuels in towns and cities combined with periods of cold weather during which little air mixing occurs has been associated with the generation of "smogs" that consist mainly of sulphur dioxide and black smoke.

In the United Kingdom today, pollution in the environment results mainly from the effluent from transport sources. The increased number of cars on our roads and increased numbers of car journeys has been a particular cause of increased pollution levels. In other cities, such as Los Angeles and Athens, air pollution is much worse than in the United Kingdom because of the higher traffic density. It is also qualitatively different in such cities, with ozone as a dominant pollutant because of the high solar radiation

Levels of the pollutants of concern in the developed world can vary substantially from country to country; even within a country, huge variations can be seen. Variations can depend on the country's infrastructure, its industries and their locations, and population demographics. Pollution does not respect borders, so pollution generated in one country can be carried to neighbouring countries and even further if the weather conditions are unfavourable.

Key pollutants

Sulphur dioxide

The main source of sulphur dioxide is the burning of fossil fuels that contain sulphur. This noxious gas is a bronchoconstrictor that irritates the upper respiratory tract in particular. People

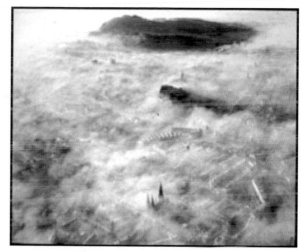
Smog over Edinburgh

Smogs

- The smog that occurred most famously in London in December 1952 saw midday London appear more like midnight, with theatres closed because the audience were unable to see the stage
- This smog episode was associated with thousands of deaths and the mortality continued to be high for weeks after the pollution episode
- As a result of such smogs, the government of the day introduced the clean air acts, which resulted in a steady decline in such pollution; air in cities in the United Kingdom is considerably cleaner now

Ambient levels of pollutants found in United Kingdom. Values are parts per billion unless otherwise specified*

Pollutant	Average concentration in United Kingdom in 2002	Very good	Good	Medium	High
Ozone	30	—	<100	100-200	>200
PM_{10} ($\mu g/ml$)	24	—	—	—	50
NO_2	20	<149	150-299	300-399	>400
SO_2	2.5	<60	60-125	125-500	>500

*Banding based on United Kingdom's Department of Health guidelines. (PM_{10} = mass per unit volume of airborne particles that are around 10 μm in diameter; NO_2 = nitrogen dioxide; SO_2 = sulphur dioxide)

Pollutants of concern throughout the developed world

- Particles
- Ozone (O_3)
- Oxides of nitrogen (NOx)
- Sulphur dioxide (SO_2)
- Volatile organic compounds (VOC)

with asthma are more sensitive to the effects of sulphur dioxide than the healthy population, as is the case for most pollutants. When a person is exposed to high enough levels of sulphur dioxide, the observed symptoms include tightness of the chest, cough, and wheeze. The increased dependency on oral breathing when people exercise impacts on the dose of sulphur dioxide delivered to that person. Oral breathing bypasses the nose, and loss of nasal scrubbing of this water soluble gas occurs. In conjunction with the increased speed of intake of respiratory gases because of exercise, this may result in a higher dose of gas being taken further into the lower respiratory system. Lung function decrements, and symptoms associated with exposure to sulphur dioxide in patients with asthma can be alleviated rapidly with the use of a β_2 adrenergic agonist medication, such as salbutamol.

Oxides of nitrogen

The oxides of nitrogen (NOx) include nitrogen dioxide (NO_2) and nitric oxide (NO). Of the two, nitrogen dioxide is potentially more harmful. In the presence of ultraviolet light and volatile organic compounds, nitrogen dioxide is converted photochemically to ozone. Nitrogen dioxide principally is derived from engine exhaust emissions, and hence in cities nitrogen dioxide can peak in the morning (because of rush hour traffic) and then ozone peaks later in the day as the nitrogen dioxide is converted progressively to ozone. These peaks, however, are influenced heavily by the meteorological conditions at a local level, with increased wind speed leading to greater dispersion. Indoors, nitrogen dioxide also is produced when cooking with gas and by tobacco smoking.

When humans are exposed to concentrations slightly higher than ambient levels in the United Kingdom, lung function is compromised, airway hyperresponsiveness increases, and patients with asthma have an increased response to allergens. In the lungs, oxides of nitrogen generate free radicals that damage and stimulate lung cells, which results in inflammation. Exposure to oxides of nitrogen also lowers resistance to respiratory infections, which is important for athletes when considering the prevalence of upper respiratory tract infections in endurance athletes. The potential for damage mediated by oxides of nitrogen in athletes is greater than in the general public because of increased ventilation rates during exercise and thus enhanced doses. Any further exacerbation of potential risks to the respiratory health of the athletes by pollutants thus must be taken very seriously, and steps should be taken to combat these problems where at all possible.

Adaptation to exposure to oxides of nitrogen has been shown at low work capacities and is evidenced by a reduced inflammatory response on re-exposure. It is not known if adaptation of the athlete in representative training or competition mode occurs, for example when working at high intensities for extended periods. The dose response of an individual to oxides of nitrogen depends on a number of factors, but short exposure to a high dose is known to be more hazardous than longer exposure to a lower dose. In cities such as Athens, oxides of nitrogen are not likely to be sufficiently elevated to effect most people, but in Beijing, for example, this pollutant is of concern.

Particulate matter

Of the main pollutants, the least is known about the effect of particulate matter (PM_{10}) on people, despite the fact that in epidemiological studies they are generally the most potent in causing adverse health effects. Reasons for the difficulty in assessing the impact of PM_{10} are the variable composition of the particulate matter and the difficulty of exposing people. It is well accepted that exposure to PM_{10} causes substantial negative

Most studies that have investigated sulphur dioxide have been conducted with very high concentrations of this pollutant. At levels normally measured in the Western developed world, this pollutant should not pose problems to the health of the general population or athletes. In more polluted locations, however—for example, Beijing—this pollutant could have a substantial impact on health and sports performance

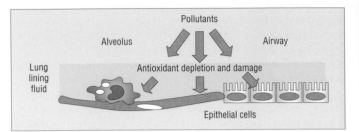

Exposure of the lung to oxidising pollutants such as particulate matter (PM_{10}) and ozone results in depletion of the antioxidant defence molecules of the lung's lining fluid. Subsequent exposure to oxidants can then impact on lung cells, resulting in loss of cilia, epithelial damage, reduced clearance of pathogens, and inflammation

In common with most pollutants, a dearth of information exists regarding the effects of oxides of nitrogen on people who work maximally or near maximally, and hence more research in this area is needed

Particulate matter (PM_{10}) denotes the mass per unit volume of airborne particles that are around 10 μm in diameter, representing particles that can be inhaled into the respiratory system

PM_{10} is a cocktail of components

Any one exposure may consist of all or some of the following:

- Carbon-based particles
- Sulphates and nitrates
- Wind blown dust
- Transition metals
- Biological components, such as bacterial endotoxin, spores, and pollen

impacts on health but it has proved much more difficult to define which components of PM_{10} are responsible for driving these health effects; this remains an intensely active field of research.

Carbon centred particles derived from combustion from traffic and industrial sources seem to be one important component. These generally fall into the nanoparticle size range (<0.1 μm). The negative effect of these particles can be further potentiated when transition metals (iron or zinc) are present.

Traffic pollution and photochemical reactions are the key sources of the sulphate and nitrate particles, which are also ultrafine. Their solubility in the lung, however, means they are unlikely to persist for long and hence have no substantial impact on health at the doses generally encountered. Wind blown dust is mainly coarse (>2.5 μM diameter), and biological components can be fine or coarse.

The size of the particles is key to the effect they have on the human. The larger particles sampled by the PM_{10} convention deposit higher up the respiratory tract—in the nose and throat. In contrast, smaller more numerous particles can deposit throughout the lungs, penetrating much further down the respiratory tract to the delicate gas exchange regions; they thus have the potential to cause more problems. The lung has a number of methods of coping with assault from particles.

Inhalation of fine particles and nanoparticles has been shown to cause acute inflammation and oxidative stress in the lungs, which leads to exacerbation of pre-existing respiratory and cardiovascular disease. Some types of experimental nanoparticles have been seen in the systemic circulation of rats within minutes of exposure—gaining access to all organ systems. Impacts of PM_{10} on the cardiovascular system occur by mechanisms that are not well understood. Increasing data show that PM_{10} increases the risk of clotting through mechanisms like increased blood viscosity. Furthermore, cardiac autonomic control is affected by exposure to PM_{10} particles; this manifests as altered heart rate variability, arterial vasoconstriction, and cardiac events. The mechanism of this effect is not clear, but it may be because of direct effect of the particles on the autonomic system eliciting a sympathetic stress response, or it could be an indirect response to inflammatory mediators released into the systemic circulation.

As with all the pollutants, the negative effects of particles on human health are well documented and accepted. The mechanism of how particle pollution, in whatever cocktail it presents itself, affects the heavily exercising athlete, however, is not known. The possibility of increased deposition and increased depth of deposition in the lungs when the human is exercising could potentially exacerbate the effect of PM_{10}. As levels of particulate exposure in Athens and Beijing are likely to have an impact on normal physiology, more investigation in this area is warranted.

Ozone

Ozone is an oxidising gas that, as mentioned previously, is generated by photochemical reactions in the atmosphere from traffic derived pollutants (NO_2 and volatile organic compounds). In terms of the human lung, ozone generates free radicals, thus depleting antioxidants in the lung lining fluid, leading to oxidative stress that damages the epithelium. This, in turn, triggers an inflammatory response that is noticeable as an increase in inflammatory neutrophils in washings from the airspaces (bronchoalveolar lavage fluid). Damage to the epithelium also results in loss of cilia, which increases susceptibility to respiratory infections. The inflammatory effects of ozone also result in decreased lung function, enhanced response to allergens, and exacerbation of asthma symptoms.

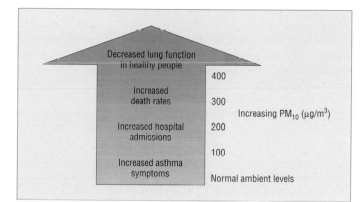

Asthmatics are sensitive to small increases in PM_{10} at levels near to those found in many cities in the United Kingdom. Little evidence exists to indicate that PM_{10} causes asthma, only that it triggers exacerbations of symptoms in people who already have this disease. Higher concentrations of PM_{10} are associated with increased hospital admissions and mortality of susceptible people. The decrease in lung function seen in normal healthy individuals only occurs at extremely high PM_{10} concentrations, which are rare in Western cities

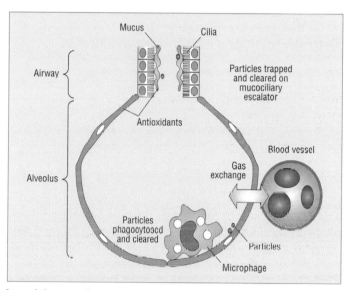

Lung defence mechanisms—when particles are deposited in the upper airways, they are then incorporated into mucus and cleared from the lung by the beating action of the cilia that transport mucus out of the airways to be swallowed. When particles deposit deeper in the respiratory parts of the lung, they are cleared by immune cells, such as macrophages. After phagocytosis, the macrophages removed the particles from the lungs via the mucociliary escalator or the lymphatic system. In addition, the lung lining fluid contains a variety of antioxidants that are designed to defend against any pollutant that induces oxidative stress

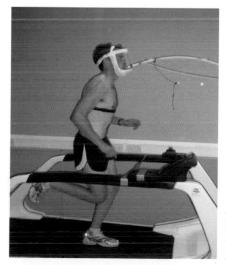

Athlete completing time trial while being exposed to ozone (100 parts per billion) via a face mask system

Ozone is the most studied of the pollutants for its effects on athletic performance.

The negative impact that ozone has on lung function seems to impair athletic performance directly. Outdoor ambient levels of ozone commonly encountered in Europe affect the lung function of athletes. Pre-exposure to ozone causes athletes to record reduced aerobic power indices and reduced performance on treadmill and cycle ergometer time trial protocols conducted in a chamber or with a face mask system.

Minimising the impact of pollution on performance

Some evidence suggests that an adaptive process takes place in people exposed to ozone. The adaptation manifests itself in the form of less severe lung function decrements and less inflammation when the individual is re-exposed to ozone than encountered after a first exposure. This is thought to result from compensatory increases in the normal antioxidant defences of the lungs. Adaptation is complex, however, and is not yet fully understood. The extent of the initial response to ozone is known to influence the extent of adaptation to subsequent exposure. In a further complication, the initial response to ozone is also very much individualised. Pre-exposing an athlete to a single concentration of ozone does not ensure adaptation to all concentrations of ozone. This could have ramifications for athletes at major sporting events in terms of their preparation and coping strategies. A pollution spike during an event, particularly on the day of competition, could negate all of the adaptive work done before the competition, as the athlete may not have adapted to such a high level of ozone. The best protocol for inducing adaptation is not clear. Adaptation has been shown to last about five days, but the length of adaptation period very much depends on the individual concerned.

As ozone, NO_x, and particles act to increase oxidative stress levels during pollution exposure, antioxidants are viewed as a possible method of reducing their impact. Antioxidants serve to mop up free radicals produced through oxidative stress mechanisms. Animal and human studies have shown that supplementation with antioxidants affords some protection against the negative affects of ozone. Severity of lung function decrements and decrements in athletic performance have decreased with the use of antioxidant supplementation, with vitamin C and vitamin E being used routinely. The protective role of antioxidants in relation to exercise performance needs further clarification before athletes consider taking this course of action. Caution should be emphasised in relation to antioxidant supplementation, in that too much antioxidant can lead to a pro-oxidant effect, possibly worsening the effects of pollution exposure.

One of the problems in trying to minimise the impact of pollution is that while the impact of individual pollutants is well documented, the impact of the complex mixture that is air pollution is not well documented. A sound understanding of the effects of a complex mixed air pollution exposure in athletes probably requires athletes to exercise in just such a pollution environment, where the effects on their performance and pulmonary function can be measured. This type of investigation is fraught with practical considerations for the researcher and, most importantly, the athlete.

Ozone concentration and lung function

The greater the concentration of ozone a person is exposed to, the larger the decrement in lung function, although the relation is not quite this simple. The duration of exposure must be taken into account, along with the minute ventilation

When these three factors are taken into account, the effective dose the person is exposed to can be calculated. Effective dose affords comparison between differing situations in terms of exercise intensity and ozone concentrations. Shorter duration exercise in a higher concentration of ozone, however, is stressed to have more pronounced effects than longer duration exercise in a lower concentration of ozone—similar to NO_2 exposure response. That is, the concentration of ozone a person is exposed to is very important in terms of the dose response

The **Department of Health in the United Kingdom** currently advises susceptible individuals, such as asthmatics and those with chronic obstructive pulmonary disease, to stay indoors during episodes of ozone pollution and to avoid strenuous exercise. Although this may be suitable for people with disease, it is hardly useful advice for athletes

In general, it would be preferable to avoid exercising in a polluted environment, but if important athletic events take place in such an environment, a period of adaptation could be advised along with a healthy intake of antioxidants through diet and possibly supplementation

More research is needed urgently to fully elaborate the interaction between the elite athlete phenotype and air pollution if rational approaches are to be developed to minimise loss of their performance

15 Diving medicine

Peter Wilmshurst

There are two types of recreational diving:

- Breath hold dive
- Scuba diving.

Scuba diving is one of the most rapidly growing participant sports in the world. Nearly 100 000 people scuba dive in the United Kingdom, with many more Britons diving only when abroad in warmer, clearer waters. Around the world, there are many millions of sport scuba divers. Most diving is an athletic pastime, but some competitive sports are undertaken by divers. For breath hold divers, these include octopush or underwater hockey, which is played at the bottom of a swimming pool, and depth and endurance record attempts. Scuba divers take part in underwater orienteering.

Breath hold diving and scuba diving take place in hostile environments and divers are at risk of illnesses unique to this sport. Divers are exposed to dangers from immersion (including hypothermia, drowning, and hypoxia), the effects of underwater pressure (including barotrauma, nitrogen narcosis, decompression illness, and toxic gas effects), and a hostile environment including trauma from boats and dangerous and venomous marine animals.

Effects of immersion

Cooling

All seas are cooler than body temperature. Water has thermal capacity and thermal conductivity 3000 and 32 times greater than air. Divers thus are cooled quickly during immersion in all but tropical waters, unless they have adequate thermal insulation from a wet suit or dry suit. Even with such insulation, hypothermia can occur if immersion is prolonged—for example if a diver is swept away from his support boat.

Hydrostatic effects

Immersion causes an increase in venous return because of the hydraulic effect of water pressure on the limbs. In warm water, this effect increases intrathoracic blood volume by up to 700 ml, which increases right atrial pressures by 18 mm Hg, cardiac output by more than 30%, and blood pressure slightly. To correct the increased central blood volume, natriuresis and diuresis are stimulated. These effects can be exaggerated by peripheral vasoconstriction from cooling. In some people, the combined effects are enough to cause cardiac decompensation and pulmonary oedema of diving and immersion.

During prolonged immersion, diuresis can produce a reduction in plasma volume so great that, when the diver is rescued and removed from the water and hydrostatic support of venous return is removed, hypovolaemic shock and sometimes death can result. To minimise the effect of removal of hydrostatic pressure, casualties who have been immersed for a prolonged period should be lifted from the water (into a boat or helicopter) with the body horizontal rather than with the legs hanging vertically down.

Other effects of immersion

Divers usually adjust their weight underwater to have neutral buoyancy. This means that they float effortlessly, but this can lead to disorientation, particularly when visibility is reduced. Even when visibility is good, differences between refraction in water and air alter the apparent size and distance of objects.

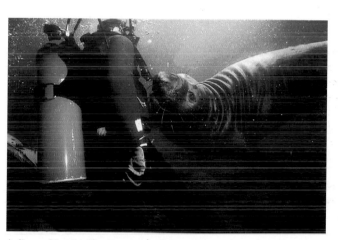

A dive to 30 m for 20 minutes puts the scuba diver at risk of nitrogen narcosis and decompression illness. The elephant seal can dive to 1 km for an hour without risk of either condition

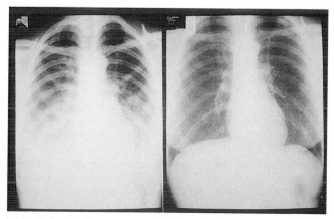

Diving induced pulmonary oedema (left) that resolved in a few hours with no treatment after diver was removed from water (right)

As a diver descends, colours are lost, initially from the red end of the spectrum. Because sound is transmitted more rapidly in water than air, distortion of noises and inability to localise the source occurs.

Effects of pressure

One needs to understand the basic properties of gases to comprehend the effects of diving on gas containing spaces and the effects of dissolved gases in the body. At sea level, atmospheric pressure is 1 bar absolute (1 standard atmosphere = 101 kPa = 1.013 bars). The weight of the atmosphere exerts a pressure that will support a column of water 10 m high. The pressure on a diver 10 m under water is 200 kPa. The volume of gas in an early diving bell full of air at sea level is halved at 10 m according to Boyle's law; at 20 m below sea level, pressure is 300 kPa absolute and the gas is compressed into one third of its original volume.

Gases dissolve in liquid with which they are in contact. Nitrogen is fat soluble, and at sea level, several litres of nitrogen is dissolved in our bodies. If the partial pressure of nitrogen is doubled (by breathing air at a depth of 10 m) for long enough for equilibration to take place, twice as many dissolved nitrogen molecules will be dissolved in the body as at sea level.

The effect of the increased partial pressure of oxygen is more complex. Oxygen is also in solution in our bodies. Doubling our inspired partial pressure of oxygen doubles the amount of oxygen in solution but does not double the amount of oxygen in the body, because a large part of the body's oxygen content is bound to oxygen carrying pigments. The haemoglobin in arterial blood is virtually saturated at an inspired partial pressure of oxygen (P_iO_2) of 21 kPa and increasing the partial pressure of oxygen has little effect on the amount of oxygen bound to haemoglobin.

Breath hold diving

An average healthy person with no special training can hold their breath for about half a minute. During the breath hold, the oxygen content of tissues decreases but the breath hold is broken because of carbon dioxide production and resulting acidosis, which stimulates the respiratory centre. With practice, a person can resist the stimulus to breathe for longer, but carbon dioxide accumulation remains the cause of release of the breath hold. The breath hold can be extended by hyperventilation immediately before the dive. Hyperventilation has little effect on the oxygen content of the body, but it expels carbon dioxide so the diver starts with a higher pH in the cerebrospinal fluid. Hyperventilation does not alter the rates of oxygen consumption and carbon dioxide production, but the low initial content of carbon dioxide in the body means that the hypoxic stimulus triggers respiration long before the pH of the cerebrospinal fluid falls enough to do so. A diver may be able to hold their breath for more than five minutes by hyperventilating on 100% oxygen. In that case, hyperventilation reduces the amount of carbon dioxide in the body but does not affect oxygen content much, but a P_iO_2 of 100 kPa considerably increases the total oxygen content.

The breath hold diver starts with a low carbon dioxide content, a high pH, and a normal oxygen tension. During descent to, say, 30 m, the pressure increases fourfold, compressing the airspaces to one quarter their surface volume (from total lung capacity of 6 l to 1.5 l—near residual volume). The partial pressures of oxygen and nitrogen in the alveoli increase fourfold and produce corresponding increases in arterial and tissue gas tensions. The alveolar carbon dioxide

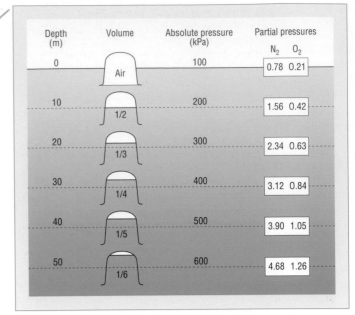

Effects of depth on partial pressures of nitrogen and oxygen

Dry air comprises about 21% oxygen, 78% nitrogen, and 1% other gases. According to Dalton's law, the partial pressure of oxygen at any depth will be 21% of the total pressure exerted by the air and the partial pressure of nitrogen will be 78% of the total pressure

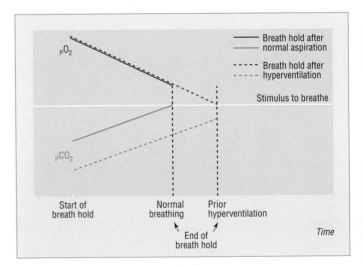

Effect of hyperventilation on breath holding

Hyperventilation before diving enables breath hold divers to stay down longer, but it is very dangerous

pressure does not change much because little carbon dioxide is present in the lungs at this point and because the body has considerable buffering capacity. During the dive, oxygen is consumed and carbon dioxide is produced. Because of the hyperventilation, the diver does not feel the need to breathe until the arterial oxygen tension has fallen to levels that stimulate the carotid chemoreceptors. As the diver ascends, hydrostatic pressure is reduced fourfold, with a fourfold reduction of the oxygen tensions in alveolar gas, arterial blood, and tissues. The rapidly falling cerebral oxygen pressure may be inadequate for consciousness to be maintained, and the diver could drown during the ascent.

> The danger of hyperventilation applies to all breath hold divers, including snorkel divers and even people swimming lengths underwater in pools. The reduction in oxygen pressure when coming to the surface from the bottom of a 2 m deep pool can be enough to cause unconsciousness—and some children have died this way

Scuba diving

Air

The most available and cheapest gas to use for scuba diving is air. It can be compressed easily. Air is mainly nitrogen, which is not inert at the high partial pressures when air is breathed at depth. This affects the function of cell membranes to cause nitrogen narcosis. Mild impairment of intellectual function may occur at only 30 m, with progressive impairment of function as the diver descends and unconsciousness at depths near 100 m.

The nitrogen that dissolves in tissues at depth also needs to be liberated on ascent or decompression. Nitrogen is highly soluble, so a large volume of gas may be involved. If the rate of decompression (ascent) is too rapid, large amounts of bubbles are liberated from the supersaturated tissues. For most air dives, the rate of ascent should be no faster than 10-15 metres per minute. For some deep or long dives, decompression stops are performed to allow gas liberation at a safe rate without excessive bubble formation in vulnerable tissues before the ascent continues. The release of small amounts of bubbles is common after innocuous dives, but too many bubbles or bubbles in the wrong place cause decompression illness. Nitrogen is also a relatively dense gas, which makes the work of breathing at 30 m twice as great as at the surface.

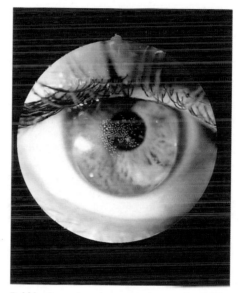

Bubbles formed on decompression may be visible in tear fluid beneath a lens

Oxygen

Several approaches have been developed to deal with the problems of nitrogen. The first was breathing 100% oxygen using a rebreathing system with a carbon dioxide absorber. The diver breathes into and out of a bellows like counterlung, with the oxygen supply topped up from a cylinder and absorption of carbon dioxide. Divers breathing pure oxygen need to carry much smaller amounts of gas, but it is associated with problems, some of which can be fatal. When a diver starts breathing oxygen from the rebreather, the diver's body contains several litres of dissolved nitrogen. The pressure gradients cause this nitrogen to pass back to the lung and into the counterlung. The oxygen is consumed, carbon dioxide is removed, and nitrogen accumulates, gradually reducing the percentage of oxygen in the counterlung. This can lead to unconsciousness. Periodic flushing of the system with pure oxygen overcomes this problem.

Prolonged breathing of a gas with a $P_iO_2 > 60$ kPa can lead to pulmonary toxicity and eventually irreversible pulmonary fibrosis, but this takes many hours or days. At a P_iO_2 greater than 160 kPa, acute oxygen toxicity can occur within minutes, causing convulsions with little or no warning. A convulsion underwater usually is fatal. The higher the P_iO_2, the greater the risk. When a person breathes air containing 21% oxygen, they are at risk of acute oxygen toxicity at depths greater than 66 m; when breathing 100% oxygen, a risk of convulsion is present at only 6 m.

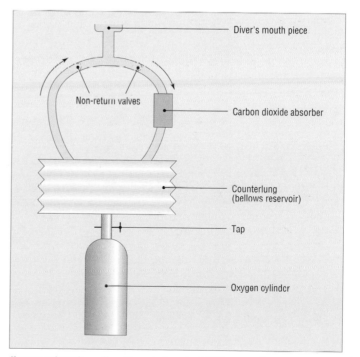

Oxygen rebreathers allow divers to breathe 100% oxygen but nitrogen accumulation can be a problem

Nitrox

Amateur divers increasingly breathe a nitrogen oxygen (nitrox) mixture, with the oxygen percentage higher than that found in air. An example would be nitrox 40, which consists of 40% oxygen and 60% nitrogen (the number always denotes the percentage of oxygen). The reduced nitrogen content compared with air increases the time the diver can stay on the bottom without getting decompression illness on surfacing. The trade off is a risk of convulsion from acute oxygen toxicity if the diver descends too deep; for nitrox 40, the depth at which this could occur would be deeper than 30 m.

Mixed gas diving

Deeper than 66 m, the gas mixture should contain a concentration of oxygen less than 21% to avoid the risk of acute oxygen toxicity. The general rule is to try to achieve a gas mixture giving a P_iO_2 of about 140 kPa. Such a reduction cannot be achieved by addition of nitrogen, however, because that would increase the risk of nitrogen narcosis and decompression illness.

Barotrauma

The gas contained within body cavities (middle ear, sinuses, and lungs) is compressed as a breath hold diver descends. For example, pain in an ear as the eardrum is pushed inwards may limit the depth achieved in a breath hold record attempt. If the diver continues the descent, the eardrum may rupture inwards, the round or oval window may rupture outwards, or haemorrhage may occur into the middle ear.

Scuba divers may also experience pulmonary barotrauma on ascent if they make a rapid ascent without exhaling adequately or have lung disease, such as a bulla, which leads to trapping of gas. Gas expands as pressure is reduced, and failure to equalise pressure can cause lung rupture. For example, during the ascent from a dive to 30 m, gas in a bulla will increase fourfold as ambient pressure reduces. If the bulla is unable to empty adequately during the ascent, it will burst and cause local lung damage, pneumothorax, surgical emphysema, or gas embolism. Gas embolism is the most common result and will have serious consequences as gas enters the pulmonary veins and passes to the left heart and hence systemic circulation. Many of the bubbles pass up the carotid arteries to cause neurological damage. If a pneumothorax occurs during ascent, the gas in the pleural space will expand as pressure is reduced (according to Boyle's law), causing a tension pneumothorax.

Decompression illness

Neurological damage can also occur if bubbles are formed during decompression. Venous bubbles are formed after many dives. Most bubbles are filtered in the pulmonary capillaries and the gas passes down the concentration gradient into the alveoli. In people with a persistent foramen ovale or other right to left shunt, paradoxical gas embolism of bubbles can occur, with venous bubbles evading the pulmonary filter and causing neurological effects. After provocative dives, so many bubbles may be liberated that the pulmonary filter is overwhelmed. Other features of decompression illness are cardiorespiratory symptoms, joint pain, and skin involvement.

Which gases should be used to dilute the oxygen on deep dives?

For a particular dive, the choice needs a compromise that takes into account the various properties of possible gases.

Helium can be used with oxygen (heliox), but helium is expensive and has a high thermal conductivity that potentiates heat loss. It can make hypothermia a serious possibility on deep dives. Helium molecules are small, so the work of breathing is low even at great depths. It is relatively insoluble in lipids, which minimises liberation of bubbles on decompression. Its insolubility means that it lacks narcotic effects.

In practice, amateur deep divers (called technical divers) usually use various mixtures of oxygen, nitrogen, and helium—called trimix. Different mixtures will be used at different stages of descent and ascent during the dive.

> Scuba divers perform manoeuvres to equalise pressures during descent and prevent occurrence of barotrauma, but equalisation may be prevented if the Eustachian tube or mouth of a sinus is blocked. Barotrauma to ears and sinuses is frequent in divers. Diving with a respiratory tract infection increases the risk of this

---

Causes of decompression illness

System affected	Right to left shunt permitting paradoxical gas embolism	Lung disease causing pulmonary barotrauma	Provocative dive profile (missed decompression stops or rapid ascent)
Neurological	Over half the cases	About a quarter of cases	Nearly a quarter of cases
Cardiorespiratory	About half the cases	About a quarter of cases	About a quarter of cases
Skin	About three quarters of cases	0	About a quarter of cases
Joint	Few if any cases	0	Almost all cases

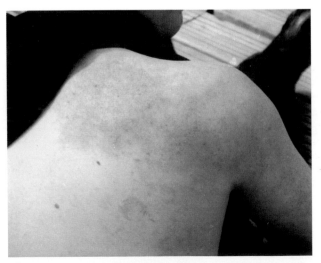

Skin bends (cutaneous decompression illness) are typically situated on the trunk and have a mottled or marbled red, blue, and purple appearance. Most are the result of paradoxical gas embolism across a shunt, but some are the result of an unsafe dive profile

Amateur sport diving

Each year in the United Kingdom, about a dozen deaths occur and more than 100 cases of serious decompression illness require recompression treatment. Most of these occur because divers fail to follow accepted safety precautions or because equipment failed or disease placed the diver at risk. Several organisations train sport divers in clubs and commercial schools. Instructors take new divers through basic theory and pool training to progressively more challenging and deeper open water dives. A trainee should be certified as competent before being allowed to undertake dives in the company of another diver without an instructor. Further training is needed before the qualified diver is able to progress to more adventurous diving.

Before anyone is allowed to start diving, and periodically when diving, they have to complete a medical declaration to ensure freedom from diseases that might predispose to incapacity in the water or diving related illnesses. The responses to the questions determine whether divers need an examination by an approved diving medical referee. Research has shown that this system of assessment does not lead to more diving accidents than having all divers examined regularly.

Lung disease in divers is a particular problem. Significant lung disease that impairs exercise performance and the ability to cope with physically demanding conditions obviously is a contraindication to diving. Asymptomatic lung disease, which does not affect exercise capacity, also is a problem. Any lung disease that causes generalised or localised gas trapping (such as emphysema, bullae, or cavities) may predispose to pulmonary barotrauma during ascent—even when the ascent rate is less than 10-15 metres per minute.

In the United Kingdom, people with mild asthma who satisfy criteria laid down by the United Kingdom Sport Diving Medical Committee may be approved to dive by a medical referee. In some countries, anyone with a history of asthma—even childhood asthma decades before—are not allowed to dive. Ironically, such countries allow smokers to dive, yet a long term heavy smoker with evidence of small airways disease on flow volume loops probably is at greater risk of pulmonary barotrauma than a mild asthmatic who has never smoked.

Medical standards also exist for non-respiratory diseases. People are advised not to dive if they have a condition that may cause incapacity in the water—for example, epilepsy and serious cardiac diseases—or predispose to diving related diseases. Hypertension predisposes to diving induced pulmonary oedema, and intracardiac shunts predispose to decompression illness. People with migraine with aura are at increased risk of decompression illness, probably because they have an increased prevalence of large persistent foramen ovale.

Surgery may have serious implications for divers. Pacemakers contain gas and are compressed by the pressure underwater. This can cause the pacemaker to fail at depth. Multiple joint prostheses and artificial limbs can alter buoyancy significantly. Seemingly innocuous drugs cannot be assumed to be taken safely by divers. Some drugs have unusual effects in divers because hyperbaric conditions may modify their actions. Schemes allow some people with disabilities to scuba dive.

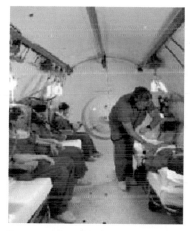
Recompression chamber

Common medical conditions that affect ability to dive

- Ear, nose and throat conditions affecting Eustachian tube function to prevent equalisation of pressure in the ear (for example, upper respiratory tract infections, allergy, enlarged adenoids)
- Sinus diseases preventing equalisation of pressure in the sinuses (for example, sinusitis, nasal polyps)
- Conditions that might lead to incapacity in the water (for example, epilepsy, diabetes, arrhythmias, coronary heart disease)
- Lung diseases that might predispose to pulmonary barotraumas or reduce exercise capacity (for example, asthma, pulmonary bullae)
- Hypertension and cardiac conditions that might predispose to immersion induced pulmonary oedema

---

Long term health hazards of diving

Diving can result in avascular necrosis of large joints (usually hip or shoulder) but the mechanism is uncertain. Uncertainty exists as to whether diving may produce other adverse long term effects, particularly in the central nervous system

---

Useful resources

Medical standards for divers
- UK Sport Diving Medical Committee (www.uksdmc.co.uk)
- British Thoracic Society Fitness to Dive Group, Subgroup of the British Thoracic Society Standards of Care Committee. British Thoracic Society guidelines on respiratory aspects of fitness for diving. *Thorax* 2003;58:3-13

Governing bodies for amateur scuba diving in the United Kingdom
- British Sub-Aqua Club (www.bsac.com)
- Scottish Sub Aqua Club (www.scotsac.com)

Further reading
- British Sub-Aqua Club. *Sport diving. The British Sub-Aqua Club diving manual.* Ellesmere Port: British Sub-Aqua Club, 2000
- Edmonds C, Lowry C, Pennefather J, Walker R. *Diving and subaquatic medicine.* London: Hodder Headline, 2002

16 Sport and disability

A D J Webborn

The achievements of athletes with disabilities remain largely unknown to most people. A high jump of nearly 2 m by a person with one leg amputated and a time of less than 1 hour 30 minutes for the wheelchair marathon show that people with disabilities are capable of considerable athletic performance.

General health

The beneficial effects of exercise are well established in relation to general health and in regard to prevention or management, or both, of specific disease processes (for example, non-insulin dependent diabetes). Participation in sport is not essential but it is important that people with disabilities are encouraged to remain physically active. People with physical disabilities are less likely to avail themselves of the beneficial effects of exercise for a variety of reasons that include cultural and social factors, facilities, and access. Evidence is accumulating to show that more physically active people with disabilities make fewer visits to doctors and have trends towards fewer medical complications and hospitalisations than sedentary counterparts. Paraplegic athletes are more successful than non-athletes in avoiding major medical complications of spinal cord injury. The message to accumulate at least 30 minutes of moderate intensity activity on at least five days of the week is equally applicable to people with and without a disability. The principles of training—that is, graded increase in duration, intensity, and frequency of activity—apply the same to people with and without a disability, but more thought may be needed as to the mode of exercise depending on the disability.

Choosing an activity or sport

In reality, people with disabilities can take part in virtually every sport available, including high risk sports such as mountain climbing, subaqua diving, and skiing. Some sports are "conventional," in that little or no modification is needed—such as swimming. Other sports may need to be adapted specifically (for example, wheelchair basketball) or developed specifically for a certain disability (for example, goalball for the visually impaired). Doctors who are counselling people with disabilities about the potential benefits of sport must establish their aims. If the aim is primarily for physical health benefits for a general health or disease modification, the difference between exercise and sport must be considered. These terms often are used interchangeably incorrectly. Sport is not always exercise and vice versa. Sport implies competition, and the physiological demands are determined by the sport—for example, wheelchair sprint racing (anaerobic) versus wheelchair road racing (aerobic) versus pistol shooting (skill). Sport may also involve trauma, which will be particularly undesirable in some conditions. Alternatively, the focus may be on socialisation and building self-esteem. Although the ability to achieve one of these aims is not necessarily exclusive of the others, the person's goals must be considered. Not all sports need be organised or competitive.

Risks of participation

In general terms, relatively few absolute contraindications exist to participation in physical activity for anybody, able bodied or

---

Recognition of athletes with disabilities

The medical profession should recognise the achievements of athletes with disabilities for two major reasons:

- To acknowledge that such people are athletes in their own right with their own sports medicine needs
- To help alter doctors' attitudes to patients with disabilities in relation to physical activity (many doctors are restrictive rather than prescriptive with exercise)

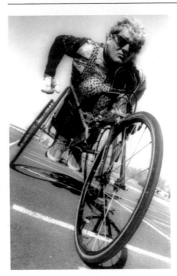

The social and psychological benefits of exercise and participation in sports are not exclusive to able bodied people, and major improvements in self-esteem of a person with a disability and social integration may result from an active lifestyle

Choice of sport is influenced by various factors

Factor	Comment
Personal preference of person	• Emphasis on enjoyment and participation in a sport that stimulates the person may be important for continued participation
Characteristics of sport	• Physiological demands, collision potential, team or individual, and coordination needs
Medical condition	• Beneficial and detrimental aspects
Conditions associated with the condition	• Although motor dysfunction initially may seem to be the major limitation to participation, an associated cardiac condition, for example may need to considered
Cognitive ability and social skills of the person	• Ability to follow rules and interact with others
Availability of facilities	
Availability of appropriate coaching and support staff (for example, lifting and handling)	
Equipment availability and cost	• As disability sport has evolved, so has the technology
	• Specialist chairs are available for sports such as tennis, rugby, and basketball
	• Although, sport specific chairs are not needed for initial participation, they do become a consideration as people develop their interest and feel more limited by their equipment

not, if the general training principles of gradual and progressive overload are applied.

History of competitive sport

Although sports associations for people with disabilities have existed since the nineteenth century, the credit for the evolution of major games for athletes with disabilities is attributed rightly to the vision and efforts of Sir Ludwig Guttmann. Guttmann was a neurosurgeon at the spinal injuries unit at Stoke Mandeville Hospital near Aylesbury in England. He introduced sport as part of the rehabilitation programme of his patients. He believed that "by restoring activity of mind and body—by instilling self-respect, self-discipline, a competitive spirit and comradeship—sport develops mental attitudes that are essential for social reintegration". The competitive spirit resulted in an archery competition on the front lawns of the hospital between 16 wheelchair competitors from the spinal unit and a disabled ex-serviceman's home in London. This was in July 1948 on the opening day of the Olympic games in London, and there started the first Stoke Mandeville games. The Athens Paralympic Games in 2004 hosted more than 4000 competitors from 130 countries with six major disability groups (see below).

Athletes are placed into different classifications according to their disability to produce fair competition. Some sports are restricted to certain disability groups—for example, judo for the visually impaired. Others allow cross-disability competition by functional assessment of sport performance as well as objective assessment by medical examination, for example, in swimming.

History of competitive sport

Historically sports for people with disabilities have developed in certain sports for certain disabled groups:

- Spinal cord lesions—congenital (through spina bifida) or acquired (through injury or disease)
- Visually impaired
- Cerebral palsy
- Amputees
- "Les autres" (the others) is a term used for people with certain disabilities that do not fit into another category—for example, those with muscular dystrophy or multiple sclerosis
- Intellectual disability
- Hearing impaired—the deaf maintain their own organisation— the Comité International Sports des Sourds (CISS) and games (the Silent Games)

Sports

In elite disability sport, the International Paralympic Committee is responsible for the organisation of the Paralympic games. The games take place two weeks after the Olympic games; this format is used for summer and winter games. Many sports other than those at the summer and winter Paralympic games are represented at world and regional championships, including lawn bowls and wheelchair dance. Each sport brings new challenges to the understanding of the sports science and medicine demands of the sport, with different injury risks through disability factors, technique, or equipment. The doctor needs to think laterally around problems that may be presented. The Paralympic games include the following sports:

- Summer—basketball, boccia, cycling, equestrianism, fencing, football, goalball, judo, powerlifting, sailing, shooting, swimming, table tennis, tennis, volleyball, wheelchair rugby.
- Winter—alpine skiing, Nordic skiing (including biathlon), ice sledge hockey.

Risks of participation

Condition	Risk
Cardiac conditions	Sudden deaths, associated with vigorous exercise or sports participation, predominantly are related to cardiac conditions For people with a disability, the doctor needs greater awareness of conditions that may have associated cardiac disease Exercise intensity is an important consideration in sport selection for people in whom cardiac anomalies may be present—for example in patients with Down's syndrome
Environmental issues	Risks of heat or cold injury may occur because of loss of autonomic function in, for example, patients with spinal cord injury Bilateral leg amputees will have reduced surface area for evaporative cooling during exercise in a hot environment
Trauma	Sports may be classified by their risk for collision potential—for example, skiing or cycling, or they may be a contact sport such as football Bone mineral density may be reduced by the nature of the patient's condition, such as in patients with osteogenesis imperfecta, or secondary to immobilisation, such as in those with paraplegia, and the risk of spontaneous fracture or fracture with minimal trauma exists The risk of atlanto-axial instability in people with Down's syndrome remains an issue of contention
Overuse injuries	Potential for overuse injury occurs in any athlete in regular training, but certain predisposing factors are likely to be more prevalent
Biomechanical factors	For example, gait in people with cerebral palsy or scoliosis in people with spina bifida
Technical factors	Coordination difficulties or restriction of movement altering correct technique
Upper limb problems	Wheelchair athletes are prone to more upper limb overuse injuries, and, in particular, degenerative changes in the shoulder have been noted in wheelchair users whether athletic or not. Good upper limb function is so important for performing activities of daily living—for example, transfers from chair to bed or bath, or propulsion—that an injury that occurs in a wheelchair athlete may have considerably different consequences on quality of life to when it occurs in an able bodied athlete

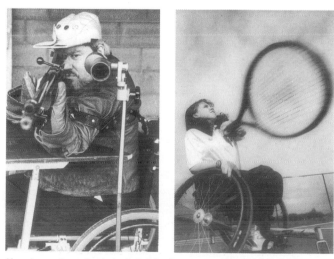

Shooting and tennis are included in the summer Paralympic games

Issues that relate to disability groups

Spinal cord lesions

The motor loss that occurs after spinal cord injury reflects the level of the lesion.

Bowels and bladder—dehydration should not occur, as this not only impairs sport performance and risks heat illness but is likely to aggravate renal calculi and infection.

Thermal regulation—loss of peripheral receptor mechanism, control of the sweating effector mechanism, and control of the ability to appropriately vasoconstrict or vasodilate the peripheral vasculature. In the cold environment the muscles will not shiver and the skin responses are not appropriate and increase the rate of heat loss.

Cardiovascular effects—a spinal cord lesion above T1 will cause absence of sympathetic cardiac innervation that produces a depressed maximal heart rate. The level of depression is determined by the intrinsic sinoatrial activity (110-130 beats per minute).

Autonomic dysreflexia—the symptoms of autonomic dysreflexia mean it is treated as a medical emergency, with treatment aimed at removing the nociceptive stimulus and reducing blood pressure with sublingual nifedipine. Reports have been made of athletes with quadriplegia intentionally inducing dysreflexia to enhance performance. This is known as "boosting" and has produced increases in simulated race times of 9.7%. Previously deemed a banned method of doping by the International Paralympic Committee, athletes suspected of being in a dysreflexic state are prohibited from competing for medical safety reasons.

Musculoskeletal injuries—data on the true incidence and type of injury in people with spinal cord lesions are limited. Chronic symptoms and symptoms of overuse in the cervical spine, thoracic spine, and shoulder and traumatic injuries to the forearm, hand, and fingers are not uncommon.

Amputees

Amputees may participate in sport with a prosthesis (for example, in sprinting and cycling) or without a prosthesis (for example, high jumping or swimming) or may compete in a wheelchair (for example, basketball). The main risks to the residual limb result from the effects of friction and compression when a prosthesis is used. Impact loading is also a concern for the residual limb, with increased ground reaction forces that may lead to degenerative change in joints higher in the kinetic chain. Technological advances in prosthetic design may reduce this loading while storing energy to facilitate propulsion.

Spina bifida

The level of motor loss determines whether people with spina bifida are ambulant or need a wheelchair for activity. Ambulant people have relatively few limitations in sport. Those with higher lesions are more prone to scoliosis that may need bracing or spinal fusion. Contractures are common, so stretching for flexibility is important for an exercise programme. Bowel and bladder function and sensory loss may be present but not the autonomic problems of the spinally injured.

Visually impaired

Visual impairment can range from complete blindness to partial sightedness that combines loss of visual acuity and field loss. The main problems specific to the disability include falls and collisions causing injury.

Factors other than level of lesion to consider in patients with spinal cord lesions

- Loss of intercostal muscle function with reduced ventilatory capacity
- Postural stability, scoliosis may require bracing for some sports
- Sensory loss and skin pressure—increased pressure and shear forces from sporting activities may increase the risk of skin ulceration
- Autonomic impairment

Thermal regulation is loss of peripheral receptor mechanism, control of the sweating effector mechanism, and control of the ability to appropriately vasoconstrict or vasodilate the peripheral vasculature

---

Usual causes and signs of autonomic dysreflexia

Causes	Signs and symptoms
• Blockage of a urinary catheter	• Severe hypertension
• Constipation	• Cerebral haemorrhage
• Urinary calculi	• Fits
• Anal fissure	• Death
• Ingrowing toenail	

A hazardous dysreflexic state is considered to be present when systolic blood pressure is ≥180 mm Hg

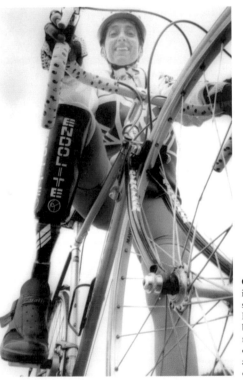

Cycling is included in the summer Paralympic games but other sports not included often have world and regional championships

---

Examples of adaptations to sports for the visually impaired

- Sound emitting ball for goalball or cricket
- Tandem cycle with sighted pilot rider
- In swimming, an assistant taps the head or shoulder of the swimmer with a soft ended pole to indicate the pool end to enable turning and finishing
- Adaptations can be made to rifles to emit an audible tone when on target
- Cross country and alpine skiing events are possible with guide skiers who give audible commands

Cerebral palsy

The three primary motor disorders that characterise the condition are spasticity, choreoathetosis, or ataxia. Hypotonic cerebral palsy is less common. At elite level, half of competitors will compete in a wheelchair while the others are ambulant.

"Les autres"

This term is used to describe people with certain disabilities that do not fit into another category. Examples include muscular dystrophies, multiple sclerosis, and short stature or limb deficiencies. To describe each of these in detail is beyond the scope of this book.

Intellectual disability

Apart from intellectual disability, other terms often used include learning disability, mental handicap, mental deficiency, and mental retardation. They all refer to the same condition. One of the most difficult problems that faces these athletes is poor perception of their sporting potential and also prejudice against them. From an organisational point of view, classification is a difficult problem in setting the level at which someone becomes eligible to participate.

Doping issues

The list of prohibited substances and methods was the same as the Olympic Movement Anti-doping Code until the adoption of the World Anti-Doping Code list in 2004. Relatively few Paralympic athletes have tested positive for banned substances and received penalties, and those who have have predominantly been involved in sports normally associated with drug misuse, such as powerlifting. A far greater number of athletes with disabilities take prescribed drugs, and attending doctors should be aware of this. Chronic pain, hypertension, and renal disease, for example, are more common in Paralympic athletes, and general practitioners often are unaware of the restrictions on prescribing for athletes.

Summary

The medical care of athletes with disabilities is a challenge for practitioners of sports medicine, which needs lateral thinking. The accepted principles of sports medicine practice need to be re-evaluated in light of the disability of the individual. A large void exists in the scientific research in sport and exercise medicine for people with disabilities that demands further attention, but the achievements of these athletes should inspire us to fill that void.

The photographs in this chapter are courtesy of Richard Bailey.

Disorders commonly associated with cerebral palsy that should be considered in sport selection

- Epilepsy
- Visual defects
- Deafness
- Intellectual impairment
- Perceptual deficits
- Speech impairment

International Paralympic Committee (IPC) and International Sports Federation for Persons with Intellectual Disability diagnostic criteria for intellectual disability

- Substantial impairment in intellectual functioning, as determined by a rating that is two standard deviations below average on an appropriate or recognised assessment instrument. (This is generally an IQ score of 75 or lower)
- Substantial limitations in adaptive behaviour as expressed in conceptual, social, and practical adaptive skills. Examples of these skills include: communication, self-care, self-direction, and social/interpersonal skills
- Intellectual disability must be evident during the developmental period. This is generally considered to be from conception to 18 years of age
- IPC rules require evidence that an athlete's disability has substantial sport related affects, which makes it impossible for the athlete to compete "on reasonably equal terms" with non-disabled athletes

---

Procedures for collecting doping samples

- To ensure integrity, athletes with visual or intellectual disabilities must have an accompanying person with them to supervise throughout the doping control process
- Sample collection methods may be adapted for athletes requiring catheters, using condom drainage or having severe disabilities, when a larger collection vessel may be used. For self-catheterisation, the athletes are allowed to use their own catheter but the bladder must first be emptied and the sample collected from the next available urine collection
- Assistance during the process may be given with the athlete's consent

---

Useful websites

- International Paralympic Association: www.paralympic.org
- Comité International Sports des Sourds: www.ciss.org
- Cerebral Palsy International Sports and Recreation Association: www.cpisra.org
- International Blind Sport Federation: www.ibsa.es
- International Sports Federation for Persons with Intellectual Disability: www.inas-fid.org
- International Stoke Mandeville Wheelchair Sports Federation: www.wsw.org.uk
- World Anti-Doping Agency: www.wada.org

Further reading

- DePauw KP, Gavron SJ. *Disability and sport*. Champaign, IL: Human Kinetics, 1995
- Fallon KE. The disabled athlete. In: Bloomfield J, Fricker PA, Fitch KD, eds. *Science and medicine in sport*. Carlton: Blackwell Science, 1995:550-1
- Goldberg B. *Sports and exercise for children with chronic health conditions*. Champaign, IL: Human Kinetics, 1995
- Webborn ADJ. Heat-related problems for the Paralympic Games, Atlanta 1996. *Br J Ther Rehab* 1996;3:429-36
- Webborn ADJ. Sports in children with physical disabilities/medical problems of disabled child athletes. In: Maffulli N, Ming Chan K, Macdonald R, Malina RM, Parker AW, eds. *Sports medicine for specific ages and abilities*. Edinburgh: Churchill Livingstone, 2001

17   Nutrition, energy metabolism, and ergogenic supplements

Clyde Williams

Athletes of this millennium have access to a far bigger range of foods than those who competed in the early Olympic Games, and yet they share many of the same misunderstandings about the influence of food on performance. One of the shared myths is that "ergogenic supplements," when found, will allow athletes to train hard, recover quickly, and compete more successfully than their rivals. The reality is that if they exist, they are probably pharmacological rather than nutritional supplements. Furthermore, in searching for such "quick fix foods," the contributions of commonly available foods to health and exercise performance are easily overlooked. The first and foremost nutritional need of athletes is a well balanced diet made up of a wide range of foods in amounts enough to cover their energy expenditure. They can then adopt nutritional strategies to ensure they can train, compete, and recover more successfully than they would if left to follow their own appetites and perceptions about what and when to eat.

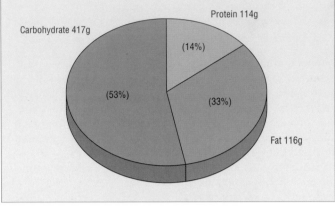

Composition of daily food intake of male distance runners

Nutrition

A well balanced diet derives at least 50% of its energy from carbohydrate containing foods, <35% from fats, and 12-15% from protein. Within the population at large, however, only endurance athletes and vegetarians have diets that match these recommendations. One of the myths that many modern athletes share with the Olympians of Antiquity is that increased meat (protein) intake helps develop strength. Mainly the strength and power athletes cling to this idea about the link between protein intake and increased strength. The reality is that athletes who undertake heavy daily training need only slightly more protein than that recommended for the general population. The daily protein requirements of most people are covered by an intake of about 1 g/kg body weight, whereas a protein intake of 1.5-1.7 g/kg is enough for athletes in heavy training. These amounts are less than the daily protein intakes of power athletes, which are often as high as 3 g/kg body mass.

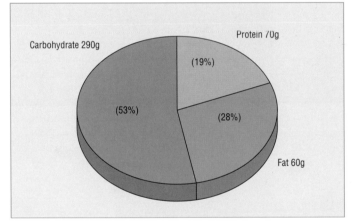

Composition of daily food intake of female distance runners

Energy balance

The amount of food consumed should be enough to cover daily energy expenditure but not be so much as to result in a substantial increase in body weight. A stable body weight is one indicator that an athlete is in energy balance—that is, that energy intake is equal to energy expenditure.

Energy balance should be assessed over several days rather than daily, however, because of the fluctuations in energy intake and expenditure. When energy intake exceeds energy expenditure as a consequence of eating even a well balanced diet, additional energy is stored as fat and carbohydrate.

"How much should I eat?" is as common a question among sportspeople as it is with less active people. The answer depends on their basal metabolic rate and their daily levels of physical activity. Basal metabolic rate is the minimum amount of energy needed to support life; it accounts for about 60% of our daily energy expenditure. It varies with age and can be estimated from body weight. One way of describing the energy cost of daily physical activity is as multiples of basal metabolic rate.

Physical activity level (PAL) =
$$\frac{\textbf{Total energy expended during 24 hours}}{\textbf{Basic metabolic rate (BMR) over 24 hours}}$$

Energy intake = energy expenditure + energy stored

For example, people who are engaged in sedentary occupations have energy expenditures about 1.55 times their basal metabolic rate, whereas, for people who participate in sports that involve prolonged heavy exercise, larger energy expenditures are needed. The top of the range of daily energy expenditures is in professional cyclists, who achieve values of 3.3 times their basal metabolic rate when racing. To maintain energy balance, therefore, these athletes must eat large amounts of energy dense foods. The energy cost of individual activities such as walking or running often are described as "mets," where an average basal metabolic rate is assumed and used as a reference value.

Many athletes want to lose body weight as a way of improving their performance because a low body weight is an advantage, such as in running, or to compete in a lower weight category as in combat sports such as wrestling. People cannot lose weight unless they are in "negative energy balance"—that is, energy intake must be less than expenditure; this is commonly referred to as "dieting." Negative energy balance can also be achieved when energy expenditure is greater than energy intake. A combination of both methods of achieving a negative energy balance is, of course, the most successful way to gain long term reductions in weight.

Popular diets only work when a negative energy balance is sustained for an extended period of time. The Atkins diet has proved popular and effective because the recommendation to eat an almost carbohydrate free diet leads to "undereating," or negative energy balance. This high protein and fat diet is not recommended for people who want or need to be physically active, because the absence of carbohydrates leads to a condition called "ketosis." High fat diets lead to reduced stores of glycogen in muscle and the liver, so the fuel for moderate to high intensity exercise is absent. Fatigue occurs earlier during such exercise in people who are on high protein and fat diets, and, furthermore, such diets do not promote optimum responses to endurance training.

Energy metabolism

The main fuels for energy production are carbohydrates and fat. Protein plays only a very minor part as a fuel during exercise in well fed people. Carbohydrate is stored in the form of a glucose polymer (glycogen) in muscle and the liver. Liver glycogen provides glucose for brain metabolism and also supplements glycogen metabolism in skeletal muscles during exercise. The average glycogen concentration in each kg of skeletal muscles is about 13 g and, in an adult man, muscle contributes about 40% to overall body mass. Therefore, the glycogen content of skeletal muscle is about 360 g and the energy yield from carbohydrate is about 4 kcal/g (16.7 kjoules/g). The energy equivalent of skeletal muscle glycogen is about 1440 kcal (6019 kjoules). Also, the adult liver, which weighs about 1.8 kg, contains about 90-100 g of glycogen, so the energy equivalent of stored carbohydrate is about 2000 kcal (8360 kjoules). About 3 g of water is stored with every gram of glycogen, so any gain in body weight after a high carbohydrate diet is not caused by the increased storage of carbohydrate alone.

Fat is stored in adipose tissue cells in the form of triacylglycerides (triglycerides) and is far more plentiful than the body's carbohydrate stores. In lean men, about 15% of their body weight is fat, whereas the value for lean women is about 20%. Complete oxidation of fat gives the equivalent of 9 kcal/g (37.6 kjoules/g), so an average 70 kg man (15% body fat) has about 94 500 kcal (about 400 000 kjoules) of energy stored as fat. The energy stored as carbohydrate thus is only 2% of the available energy stored as fat.

The metabolic degradation of fat and carbohydrate produces ATP, described as the "energy currency of life." Almost every physiological process that needs energy uses ATP, and, because it is not stored in large quantities, it has to be

In the Tour De France, professional cyclists have daily energy intakes of about 6500 kcal (27.17 MJ); this increases to about 9000 kcal (37.6 MJ) during the mountain section of the race. Their average daily energy intake is about double that of active healthy people (2500-3000 kcal)

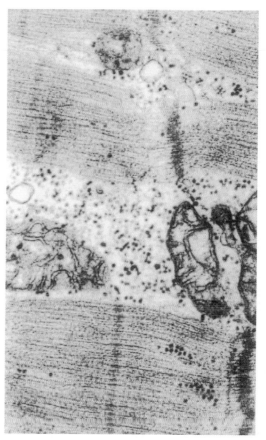

Electron photomicrograph of human muscle. The sample, obtained by percutaneous needle biopsy, was taken before exercise to fatigue. The black dots are the glycogen granules dispersed between the myofibrils and mitochondria. Clear droplets of triglycerides are also visible although not as abundant as the glycogen granules

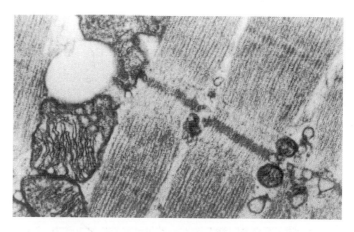

Electron photomicrograph of human skeletal muscle. The sample, obtained by percutaneous needle biopsy, was taken when the subject fatigued after two hours of cycling. The absence of glycogen granules provides supportive evidence for the strong association between glycogen depletion and fatigue

resynthesised rapidly. At rest, resynthesis of ATP is achieved mainly by oxidation of fat, with only a minor contribution from metabolism of carbohydrate.

Oxidation of fat and carbohydrate occurs in mitochondria, which are like small cells within cells. The capacity for aerobic metabolism relates directly to the number of mitochondria in each muscle fibre. Muscle comprises two populations of fibres:

- Type 1: slow contracting, slow fatiguing fibres that are generally rich in mitochondria
- Type 2: fast contracting, fast fatiguing fibres with relatively few mitochondria.

As we move from rest to exercise, ATP is used more rapidly to cover the energy demands of working skeletal muscles. During onset of exercise, the rate of ATP production from oxidation of fat and carbohydrate is too slow to match the rate at which ATP is used. This is largely a result of initial adjustments of the cardiovascular system to increased demands for oxygen delivery. The oxidative contribution of the fat and carbohydrate to ATP production is, therefore, temporarily inadequate. Fortunately, mechanisms are in place to cover this temporary energy deficit, otherwise we would not have the ability to sprint or change running speed as and when the occasion demands. We cope because muscle has a high energy compound called phosphocreatine, which has three times more potential energy than ATP. In energy demanding cellular processes, ATP is reduced to ADP (adenosine diphosphate). Phosphocreatine rapidly converts ADP to ATP to allow the contractile activity in skeletal muscle to continue, during which time the contributions to ATP resynthesis from fat and carbohydrate increase gradually.

Carbohydrate metabolism helps cover some of the energy deficit at the start of exercise, because the early steps in the degradation of muscle glycogen do not require oxygen. This is described as the anaerobic degradation of glycogen, which provides three ATP molecules rather than the 38 ATP molecules that result from complete degradation. This smaller number of ATP is produced rapidly, however, and so helps phosphocreatine quickly to replace the ATP used by working skeletal muscles. Anaerobic or non-oxidative production of three ATP molecules is accompanied by formation of lactic acid (or, more accurately, lactate and hydrogen ions).

After several minutes of submaximal exercise, oxygen demand is met by oxygen delivery and ATP is produced by the oxidation of fat and carbohydrate. The relative contributions are dependent, however, on a number of physiological conditions. The first is the exercise intensity relative to the person's maximum capacity for oxygen consumption ($\dot{V}O_{2max}$). At low relative exercise intensities ($<50\% \ \dot{V}O_{2max}$), fat is the main fuel with only a minor contribution from carbohydrate metabolism. As exercise intensity increases, carbohydrate metabolism has a greater contribution, and fatigue occurs when stores of muscle glycogen are used up. Carbohydrate used during exercise is not confined to muscle glycogen, however, because blood glucose derived from the liver also contributes to muscle metabolism (but mainly during later stages of prolonged exercise).

Long chain fatty acids are mobilised from adipose tissue cells and transported in loose combination with plasma albumin to working muscle. Here, they are taken up and oxidised in mitochondria or stored as intramuscular triglycerides. Intramuscular triglycerides contribute to muscle metabolism, especially when the delivery of plasma fatty acids is less than the capacity of muscle to oxidise them. Fat and carbohydrate act in concert with phosphocreatine to cover the ATP needs of skeletal muscle. The relative contributions of these two fuels are also influenced by the training status of the person and the composition of the last meal.

Short term and long term reductions in energy intake

To lose 1 kg of body mass, a person must achieve a negative energy balance equivalent to about 7000 kcal. This could be achieved by reducing daily energy intake by 1000 kcal for a week; however, this severe reduction in food intake would need a great deal of discipline and may undermine the ability of an athlete to train successfully

A longer term approach is more likely to achieve success without compromising the capacity of an athlete to continue to complete heavy training than a rapid reduction in energy intake. A reduction in daily energy intake of 250 kcal for one month would bring about the desired body weight change of 1 kg. It is sustainable and so an athlete could go onto lose a greater amount should it be required

One note of caution is that when body mass is reduced by 1 kg only about three-quarters of the weight loss is fat, the rest is lean tissue

---

Type 1 fibres mainly resynthesise ATP by aerobic metabolism of fat and carbohydrate. In contrast, type 2 fibres (sprint fibres) rely almost entirely on anaerobic degradation of glycogen to complement phosphocreatine (see below) in resynthesising ATP during exercise

---

The appearance of lactate in the blood often is interpreted wrongly as energy production in the absence of cellular oxygen rather than as reflecting the differential rates of aerobic and anaerobic production of ATP

Oxidation of long chain fatty acids produces about 140 ATP molecules, whereas oxidation of glycogen produces only 38 ATP molecules

---

Endurance training and energy consumption

Endurance training increases the number of capillaries around each of the type 1 fibres and their mitochondrial density. The consequence of this adaptation is that, during submaximal exercise, the endurance trained individuals will use more fat to cover their energy expenditure than the less well trained. As a result, the rate of glycogen degradation will be slower and so endurance capacity will increase

---

Brief high intensity exercise and energy consumption

During brief high intensity exercise, such as sprinting, the limiting factor is not glycogen depletion but probably the widespread cellular effects of a decrease in muscle pH. The capacity to perform repeated maximum sprints depends not only on delaying a severe reduction in muscle pH but also on the muscle's ability to rapidly resynthesise phosphocreatine between sprints. When the intensity of each sprint is slightly less than maximal, after many more sprints, depletion of muscle glycogen again becomes the limitation to further exercise. In a multiple sprint sport, such as soccer, the players with low levels of glycogen in muscle run less than the players with more adequate stores of glycogen

Two menus for high carbohydrate diets

Meal	Menu 1	Menu 2
Breakfast	Four wholewheat biscuits Semi-skimmed milk Two crumpets with honey Orange juice Tea or coffee (preferably decaffeinated)	Baked beans on thick sliced toast Three slices of toast Low-fat spread (thinly spread) Orange juice Tea or coffee (preferably decaffeinated)
Mid-morning snack	Malt loaf Low-fat spread (thinly spread) Diet squash (1 pint)	Two digestive biscuits Banana Low-fat milkshake
Lunch	French bread Lean ham Reduced fat cheddar cheese Low-fat spread (thinly spread) Pickles Low-fat rice pudding Pear Diet squash and water	Wholemeal bread roll Lean beef Low-fat spread (thinly spread) Tomato, lettuce, and cucumber Packet of "French Fries" crisps Low-fat fruit yoghurt Diet squash and water
Mid-afternoon snack	Apple and banana Diet squash or water	Currant bun Tea or coffee (preferably decaffeinated)
Dinner	Roast chicken with mushrooms, onions, peas, and mixed vegetables (stir fried in a sweet and sour sauce) Boiled basmati rice Swiss roll and vanilla dairy ice-cream Tea or coffee (preferably decaffeinated)	Pasta with lean ham, mushrooms, onion, and cheese sauce (made with semi-skimmed milk and a cheese sauce packet mix) Bread roll Bread and butter pudding Tea or coffee (preferably decaffeinated)
Supper	Fruit and fibre containing cereal Semi-skimmed milk Diet squash and water	Five gingernut biscuits Low-fat hot chocolate
Energy		
Total (kcal)	2944	2804
Protein (%, g)	19 (183)	16 (112)
Fat (%)		22
Carbohydrate (%)	65	62

Nutritional strategies

Before exercise

Recognition of the central role carbohydrate plays in energy metabolism during exercise means it is not surprising that nutritional strategies have been developed to increase muscle glycogen stores before exercise. The most effective and acceptable method of "carbohydrate loading" is to decrease training 3-4 days before competition and increase consumption of carbohydrate containing foods in each meal. A daily intake of about 9-10 g/kg body weight of carbohydrate is enough to increase muscle and liver glycogen stores prior to competition. Furthermore, a high carbohydrate meal eaten 3-4 hours before competition also helps top up glycogen stores. The nature of the carbohydrate, however, will influence the amount of fat metabolism before and during exercise. A meal containing carbohydrates with a high glycaemic index will increase plasma glucose and insulin concentrations and, as a result of the elevated insulin concentrations, will inhibit fatty acid mobilisation from adipose tissue cells. The decreased availability of fatty acids will be covered by an increase in carbohydrate metabolism in skeletal muscles, with some contribution from intramuscular triglycerides.

Ideal pre-exercise meals provide enough carbohydrate to top up fuel stores in the liver and muscle without causing too severe a reduction in the rate of fat oxidation during subsequent exercise. Recent research suggests that a meal containing carbohydrates with a low glycaemic index eaten three hours before exercise leads to a greater rate of fat oxidation and endurance capacity during prolonged running than a high pre-exercise meal containing carbohydrates with a high glycaemic index.[1] The greater benefit of pre-exercise meals that contain carbohydrates with a low glycaemic index also extends to

> A pre-exercise meal that contains carbohydrate with a low glycaemic index does not depress fatty acid mobilisation or utilisation to the same extent as meals containing carbohydrate with a high glycaemic index

Low glycaemic index carbohydrate diet

Breakfast
70 g All Bran or porridge
200 ml skimmed milk
Half an apple
Half a tin of peaches (in natural juice)
Pot of low fat yoghurt
1 glass of apple juice

Lunch
140 g wholewheat pasta
100 g grilled turkey breast
150 g tomato based pasta sauce
1 glass of apple juice
1 pear

Snack
1 pot of low fat fruit yoghurt
1 apple
Handful of nuts

Dinner
1 tin of taco beans
2 wheat tortillas
40 g low fat grated cheese
Lettuce and tomato
1 glass of fresh orange juice

Energy 2800 kcal of which carbohydrate 70%, protein 15%, fat 15%

recovery from exercise. A "recovery diet" that contains carbohydrates with a low glycaemic index eaten during the 24 hours after prolonged running results in a greater endurance capacity the next day than a recovery diet that consists mainly of carbohydrates with a high glycaemic index.

During exercise

Dehydration can cause fatigue during prolonged exercise, even before stores of glycogen in muscle are depleted. Drinking well formulated solutions that contain carbohydrate and electrolyte solutions (for example, sports drinks) throughout exercise helps prevent severe dehydration and contributes to carbohydrate metabolism in working muscles; this delays the onset of fatigue. Sports drinks that provide carbohydrate at a rate of 30-50 g/hour are effective in increasing endurance performance.

After exercise

Speed of recovery from exercise depends on how quickly muscle glycogen can be replaced and fluid balance restored. Muscle glycogen resynthesis is most rapid immediately after exercise, so a solution that contains carbohydrate and electrolyte (or eating foods containing carbohydrates with a high glycaemic index) drunk after exercise will produce the maximum rate of glycogen resynthesis. Delaying the consumption of carbohydrate for 2-3 hours after exercise reduces the rate of glycogen resynthesis and delays the return of endurance fitness. When an athlete is attempting to recover within 24 hours, food intake must be prescribed because ad libitum intake will not provide enough carbohydrate to replace muscle glycogen or restore energy balance.

Nutritional (ergogenic) supplements

Unfortunately, too many sportspeople are vulnerable to advertising claims that supplements enhance performance. The most popular nutritional supplements are described below. Many manufacturers of others make claims without any supporting evidence, and these have not been included here.

Vitamins and minerals

Supplementation with vitamins and minerals is common practice among many sportspeople, despite no good evidence to show that performance is enhanced after a period of supplementation in a person who eats a well balanced diet with additional vitamins and minerals. The assumption that all athletes eat a diet containing a wide range of foods that provide enough energy to cover their energy expenditure is not always true. People who participate in sports with strict weight categories generally try to compete in a weight class lower than their normal training weight.

Amino acids

In addition to eating foods that contain extra protein, many strength athletes also supplement their diets with amino acids, especially those such as arginine, which stimulate increased release of growth hormone. The growth hormone releasing effect of these amino acids is far less than that produced by exercise alone, however, and too many strength athletes, and their coaches, mistakenly continue to extol the performance benefits of supplementation with amino acids.

Branched chain amino acids also have been suggested as a way of delaying "central fatigue." The central fatigue concept proposes that the rise in plasma free tryptophan during prolonged exercise increases levels of serotonin—one of the brain's neurotransmitters—which in turn decreases the drive to continue exercising. Branched chain amino acids (valine,

---

Note of caution about "over drinking"

Athletes should try to relate their drinking to their rate of sweating—that is, when sweating heavily then larger volumes of fluid intake should be ingested than when sweat rates are low. Simply drinking water in excess of sweat rates could dilute the sodium concentration in the blood and lead to hyponatraemia and ultimately collapse

---

Carbohydrate consumption after exercise

- Optimum amount of carbohydrate is 1 g/kg body weight, which is achieved by drinking about a litre of a sports drink containing 6 to 7% carbohydrate
- Consuming 50 g of carbohydrate every hour until the next meal, however, seems to be a more practical recommendation
- Overall carbohydrate intake during the recovery over a 24 hour period should be equivalent to about 10 g/kg body weight

---

Popular nutritional supplements

- Vitamins
- Minerals
- Amino acids
- Creatine

Low energy intakes and high energy expenditures have the potential for nutrient deficiency. This is particularly true for women, who must pay particular attention to their intake of iron, calcium, and folic acid

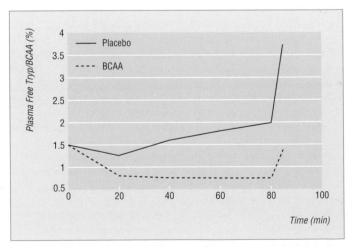

Ratio of plasma concentrations of free tryptophan to branched chain amino acid (BCAA) during prolonged exercise after ingestion of BCAA and placebo. Adapted from Blomstrand et al. *Acta Physiol Scand* 1997;159:41-9

leucine, and isoleucine) cross the blood-brain barrier by the same carrier mechanism as tryptophan. Increasing the plasma concentration of branched chain amino acids is hypothesised to competitively inhibit tryptophan's transport across the blood-brain barrier and avoid large increases in serotonin. Ingestion of branched chain amino acids during prolonged exercise increases plasma concentrations of branched chain amino acids and reduces the ratio of free tryptophan to such amino acids. The rate of perceived exertion is reduced, but endurance performance does not improve with such supplementation.

Bicarbonate loading

During brief high intensity exercise, such as sprinting, a rapid rate of glycogen degradation is accompanied by an increase in accumulation of lactate and hydrogen ions. The resulting acidity in muscle cells is associated with onset of fatigue. The blood's increased capacity for buffering encourages transfer of hydrogen ions out of the muscle cells and so helps restore the pH more quickly to pre-exercise values. Ingestion of a bicarbonate solution increases the athlete's capacity to perform high intensity exercise for short periods of time. For example, bicarbonate loading substantially improves performance times of non-elite runners in 400 m, 800 m, and 1500 m races. The dose of bicarbonate is 300 mg/kg body mass taken an hour or more before exercise. Higher doses cause gastrointestinal disturbances and, in some people, nausea and diarrhoea.

Creatine

In multiple sprint sports, the rate of ATP resynthesis is more important than the capacity for energy production. Rapid resynthesis of ATP occurs as a result of contributions from the degradation of phosphocreatine and glycogenolysis. Performance during a series of maximum sprints separated by recovery periods of no more than 30 seconds decreases because not enough time is available for resynthesis of phosphocreatine. Creatine supplementation before exercise delays this decrease in performance by increasing resynthesis of phosphocreatine. The main source of creatine is foods that contain meat or fish. Creatine monohydrate is the supplement used, however, and 1 g is equivalent to the creatine content in 1 kg of fresh meat. In laboratory studies, the effective dose of creatine is 20-30 g/day for 5-6 days. Creatine supplementation at this level increases the pre-exercise phosphocreatine concentration. Lower doses of creatine also seem to influence performance during repeated sprints when recovery between sprints is longer than 60 seconds.

Caffeine

Consumption of caffeine in the form of strong coffee or in tablet form was suggested as a way of increasing mobilization of fatty acids from fat cells. Increased availability of fatty acids should then increase the amount of fat metabolism in skeletal muscles and so reduce the contribution of the limited stores of glycogen in muscle to energy production. Caffeine, however, has a much more powerful effect on the central nervous system than on fat cells per se. Caffeine's impact on the brain results in improvements in performance after caffeine ingestion rather than a caffeine induced increase in fatty acid mobilisation. Even relatively small doses of caffeine have a substantial ergogenic effect. As little as 9 mg caffeine per kilogram of body mass improves endurance capacity without increasing urine concentration to higher than the former International Olympic Committee's limit of 12 mg/l. Although the ban on caffeine intake has been removed by the International Olympic Committee, great care should be taken when caffeine is used as an ergogenic aid because "more doesn't mean better," from a health perspective.

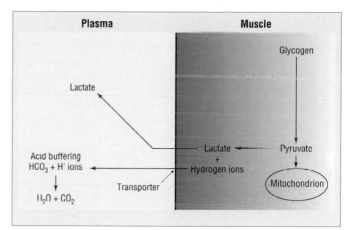

Bicarbonate metabolism. The mechanisms by which an increase in plasma bicarbonate concentration increases the translocation of hydrogen out of the muscle cell

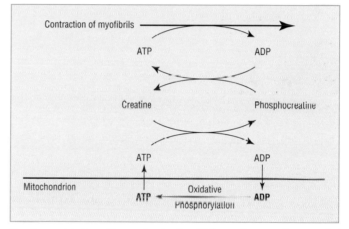
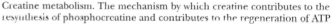

Creatine metabolism. The mechanism by which creatine contributes to the resynthesis of phosphocreatine and contributes to the regeneration of ATP

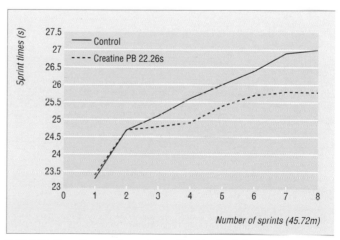

Influence of creatine supplementation (9 g/day for 5 days) on performance during sprint swimming (8 × 45.72 m (50 yards)) at intervals of 90 seconds. (PB = personal best). Adapted from Peyrebrune M et al. *J Sports Sci* 1998;16:271-9

Summary

Apart from appropriate training, a high carbohydrate diet and adequate fluid intake are the essential elements for successful preparation for participation in, and recovery from, sport and exercise. Strategic supplementation of some nutrients, such as creatine, may benefit participants in multiple sprint sports.

Further reading

- Maughan R, ed. *Nutrition in sport. Encyclopaedia of sports medicine (IOC Medical Commission publication)*. Oxford: Blackwell Science, 2000
- Maughan R, Gleeson M, Greenhaff P, eds. *Biochemistry of exercise and training*. Oxford: Oxford University Press, 1997
- Burke L, Collier G, Hargreaves M. Glycemic index—a new tool in sports nutrition. *Int J Sport Nutr* 1999;8:401-15

1 Wu CL, Nicholas C, Williams C, Took A, Hardy L. The influence of high-carbohydrate meals with different glycaemic indices on substrate utilisation during subsequent exercise. *Br J Nutr* 2003;90:1049-6

18   Diet, obesity, diabetes, and exercise

Patrick Sharp

Obesity

Prevalence

Adults

A glance at the graph showing prevalence of obesity is all that is needed to highlight the problem we face with respect to obesity in developed societies. The figures from the Health Survey for England and Wales indicate a steady increase in the percentage of adults aged over 16 years—men and women alike—who have a body mass index (BMI) > 30. BMI is calculated by weight (kg)/(height (m)²). The worrying feature of the data is that not only have more than 20% of the adult population reached the classical cut off for a definition of obesity, but as yet there is no sign that the increasing trend is levelling off. Similar findings are reported in all developed societies, the growing tendency to obesity is most acute in developing countries, where rates are increasing most rapidly.

Children

Traditionally, obesity has been thought of as a problem in adults; however, an increasing body of information relates to overweight in children. In the United States in 2000, 22% of preschool children were classified as overweight and 10% as obese. Data from the National Longitudinal Survey of Youth, a study of child health in the United States, shows marked similarities with the trends in increasing obesity in adults. Similar results have been found in the United Kingdom. The Health Survey for England in 2001 reported that 8.5% of children aged 6 years and 15% of those aged 15 years were obese. A worrying trend for the increase in obesity to be more marked in certain ethnic groups is not unique to the United States and needs to be investigated further to ascertain the cause and devise solutions.

Causes

Debate is ongoing as to the cause of increased rates of obesity in industrialised societies: increased food intake or lack of exercise. Much has been written about high fat, high salt diets encouraging increased food intake; however, the Expenditure and Food Survey from the Department for Environment, Food and Rural Affairs estimates per capita daily calorie intake in England and Wales to have remained steady at 1900-2000 calories between 1996 and 2002. The National Food Survey, which has been documenting qualitative and quantitative changes in food intake in the United Kingdom for many years, indicates that daily calorie intake has been falling. Such surveys could be argued to underreport calories consumed out of the home and "on the move," but accepting the data as they are, and plotting changes against data on BMI from the Health Survey for England and Wales, it is not possible to conclude that an increase in food intake is the problem.

By contrast, any marker of physical inactivity, such as hours of television watching or car ownership and use show a progressive rise. The conclusions are inescapable. Most of the population is in positive energy balance, with energy intake exceeding expenditure. The problem is highlighted with respect to children, as data from the United States show a progressive decline in physical activity, to the point that certain children take part in no exercise by the age of 7 years. This must be a factor in the increased prevalence of obesity in this age group, and is

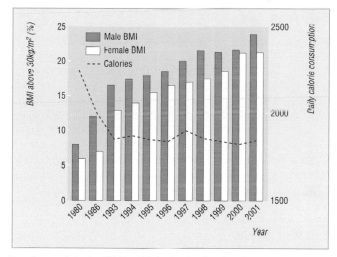

Prevalence of obesity (BMI > 30) in England and Wales superimposed with daily calorie intake per head. Data from Health Survey for England and Wales, Expenditure and Food Survey, and National Food Survey

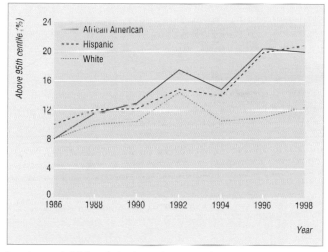

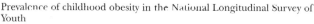

Prevalence of childhood obesity in the National Longitudinal Survey of Youth

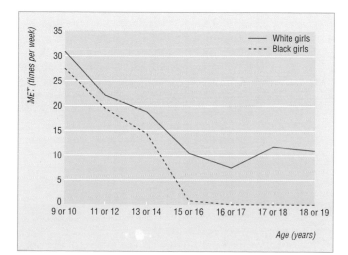

Physical activity in white and black girls by age. Adapted from Kimm SY et al. *N Engl J Med* 2002;347:709-15. (MET = metabolic equivalent)

certainly an issue that needs urgent attention. Those who argue that genetic differences account for the increased rates of obesity in certain ethnic groups should take note of differences in physical activity in different societies, which show that cultural differences are equally important and need to be addressed.

Diabetes

Epidemiology

Projected changes in prevalence of diabetes in Europe and worldwide are impressive. Although such figures might seem fanciful, they are, in fact, based on some very simple and robust calculations. For each country in the study, future population growth, and hence population numbers at any particular time, were calculated. Future prosperity was calculated on the basis of projected gross national product. The number of people with diabetes was derived from data from epidemiological studies in similar populations. To date, the projections seem to be holding true and indicate why urgent action is needed to reduce the incidence of type 2 diabetes.

Obesity and diabetes

The commonly used cut off for obesity (BMI = 30) may seem harsh to many, given that obesity is common as discussed above. The literature, however, is quite uncompromising in demonstrating the adverse effects of obesity. The relation between mortality and body weight is a J shaped curve, with a sharp increase when the BMI is more than 30; however, the upswing starts at a BMI of 25. The risk of coronary artery disease increases 3.3-fold when people with a BMI greater than 29 are compared with those with a BMI of 21. Control of obesity has been estimated to eliminate hypertension in 48% of cases in a white population. Given the hard cut off points for a definition of diabetes, the relation between body weight and diabetes has been well defined. Data show a steady increase in the relative risk of diabetes with increasing body weight. The relation is continuous, but the rapid increase occurs in people with a BMI ≥ 30. Of course, obesity could be a marker of insulin resistance rather than the cause, but studies of exercise in prevention, as discussed below, suggest that this is not the case.

Children

For many of us who deal with patients with diabetes, a very apparent and worrying trend is seen in the prevalence of type 2 diabetes in young people. Traditional teaching was that type 2 diabetes was a disease of older people, and this was reflected in the now obsolete term "maturity onset diabetes." In recognition of changing patterns of disease, the term has now been scrapped in favour of the less judgmental terminology "type 2 diabetes." Literature in the 1980s reported on the phenomenon of maturity onset diabetes of the young, when such cases were rare. Nowadays, young adults commonly present with diet or tablet responsive diabetes in young adulthood.

In one study, overweight in young people was associated with all classical vascular risk factors—an adverse lipid profile and increased systolic and diastolic blood pressure.[1] Obese children have an increased incidence of diabetes, with the end result that one-third of all new cases of diabetes in those aged 10-19 years could be classified as type 2 diabetes.

Exercise

Studies on exercise and weight loss

Given the publicity surrounding the adverse effects of obesity, and the current (perhaps paradoxical) fashion for "thin is beautiful," many people are motivated to lose weight. One of

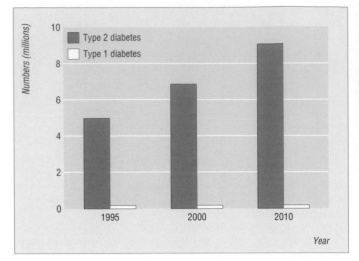

Projected number of people with diabetes in Europe. Source: *Diabet Med* 1997;14:S33

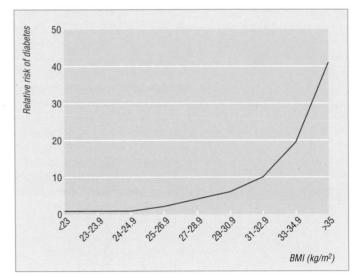

Relative risk of diabetes by body mass index. Colditz GA et al. *Ann Intern Med* 1995;122:481-6

> Young adults with diet or tablet responsive diabetes have all the risks for diabetes previously thought to be the preserve of older adults

> Prevalence of obesity in the young is increasing rapidly, and the young are not spared the metabolic consequences of premature weight gain

Incidence of type 2 diabetes in children*

- Among Japanese children, the incidence of type 2 diabetes now is reported as 7.2 per 100 000 per year—a figure close to the reported incidence of type 1 diabetes
- Among obese youngsters, 25% of those aged 4-10 years had impaired glucose intolerance; the corresponding figure in those aged 11-18 years was 21%
- In the older age group, however, 4% had overt diabetes

*Adapted from Pinhas-Hamiel O et al. *J Pediatr* 1996;128:608

the first ports of call in achieving this is exercise. Those involved in advising in such matters must be aware of the literature on the subject. Meta-analysis of published studies of walking and running indicated that weight loss of about 0.09 kg per week was achievable. Results have been fairly consistent on this topic, and subsequent studies involving programmes of running or cycling have shown weight loss of 0.1 kg per week. More detailed studies of body composition have confirmed that loss of fat mass may actually be double this but is masked by the increase in muscle mass. Nevertheless, individuals should be advised of exactly the amount of weight they might expect to see on the scales by this means. Unfortunately, 0.1 kg per week can be lost in the week to week variation in body weight, and many people, expecting a quick return, can be discouraged by lack of rapid apparent results.

Given the concern surrounding the growing incidence of obesity in the United Kingdom, a critical review of the evidence surrounding strategies to reduce weight was published recently.[2] The disparate nature of the data and different methods used make it hard to draw firm conclusions other than that we need to continue to build on this database of practical interventions to treat diabetes and obesity. Evidence does seem to show, however, that strategies that involve at least one parent are more effective in encouraging weight loss in young children than those that involve schools alone. In adolescents, the same may not be true. Dietary restriction is also noted as a more effective means of losing weight than exercise alone—at least in the short term—although this does not take into account the other health benefits of exercise programmes.

Studies of preventative effect of exercise on diabetes

Given the projected epidemic of diabetes, that many studies have looked at the effects of exercise on prevention and treatment is unsurprising. In the early 1980s, small scale studies first showed that exercise programmes could prevent worsening of glucose tolerance and development of assays to measure insulin showed that such changes were associated with reductions in insulin levels. In other words, inactivity and obesity were associated with raised insulin levels as a function of insulin resistance. Exercise was seen to reverse this effect.

On the back of such observations, larger clinical studies were launched. In a study of over 21 000 subjects followed for five years, the incidence of diabetes was related to habitual levels of exercise.[3] In those who exercised five times a week, the incidence of diabetes was lower than in those who exercised only once a week (214 vs 369 per 100 000 person years). When body weight was factored in, the biggest decrease in the onset of diabetes was found in those with the highest BMI. These results were very similar to those from a study of nearly 600 men, which documented the incidence of diabetes in relation to exercise level and BMI.[4] In this group, people who exercised more had a lower rate of onset of diabetes; however, this effect was greatest in those with a BMI > 26.

More recent studies have focussed on the issue of preventing diabetes. A rewarding study group in this context comprises people with impaired glucose tolerance. People with a two hour glucose value of 8-11 mmol/l from a 75 glucose tolerance test are classified in the grey area of impaired glucose tolerance. In more recent diagnostic criteria for diabetes, those with fasting glucose of 6-7 mmol/l are classified as having impaired fasting glucose tolerance. These groups are valuable because they have a fast rate of progression to overt diabetes, so interventions can be assessed within a short time frame.

In a study from the Northern Chinese city of Da Qing, a large scale screening programme followed 530 people with impaired glucose tolerance for six years. Study participants were

> More extreme exercise regimens, such as in military recruits and others engaged in daily and prolonged exercise programmes, have shown weight loss of 0.6-1.8 kg per week, but it would not be realistic to offer this figure to weight loss aspirants

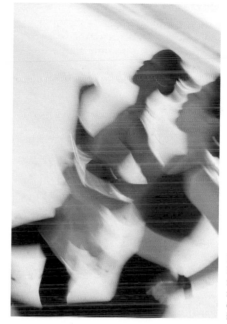

Exercise as a means of losing weight is not a rapid solution but rather should be considered as a change in lifestyle

> In adults, workplace exercise programmes are effective, although results depend on energy expended and enthusiasm

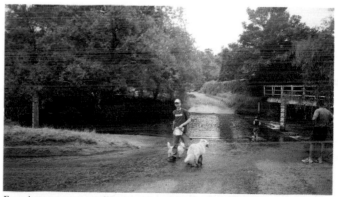

Exercise programmes that are not sustainable should be discouraged, and people should be advised to build exercise into their lives in a long term fashion

Study groups in Da Qing impaired glucose tolerance study

- People who were advised on a healthy eating diet
- People who were advised on increasing their exercise levels and taught exercises
- People who were advised on diet and exercise
- People who were given general information only (controls)

divided into four groups.

In the control group, the progression to diabetes was 67.7% over 6 years compared with 41.1% in those in the exercise group. In fact, the exercise group fared better than those who received any other intervention.

In a larger study in the United States, remarkably similar results were obtained. More than 3000 patients were assigned to one of three groups consisting of standard advice, standard advice plus metformin (850 mg a day), or an intensive lifestyle modification programme that included brisk walking for at least 150 minutes a day. Incidence of diabetes was 58% lower in the intensive intervention group than the routine care group, with metformin treatment between the two groups.

The results of such studies confirmed the effectiveness of an exercise programme in improving insulin sensitivity and in preventing the onset of diabetes in susceptible people. The data presented above, which suggest an "epidemic" of type 2 diabetes in the next two decades, give a message that is hard to ignore.

Exercise in people with diabetes

A number of studies have assessed the effects of exercise in people with existing diabetes. An exercise programme seems to reduce the haemoglobin $A1_c$ by 1%, which is similar to the benefit seen with many pharmacological interventions and certainly is enough of an improvement to prevent many of the future complications of diabetes.

Type 1 diabetes

As a general principle, patients with type 1 diabetes should be encouraged to lead as normal a life as possible, despite the need to take insulin and monitor blood glucose. By extension, they should also be allowed to participate in any sporting activity they wish. Certain sports, such as deep sea diving, may be difficult, but as one patient pointed out, "it is possible to eat carbohydrate at 50 m; it just doesn't taste very nice."

In people who take insulin and exercise on a regular basis, it is advisable to move to an insulin regimen in which a long acting insulin is taken at bedtime and short acting insulin is taken with each meal (a "basal bolus regimen"). This allows much more flexibility in adjusting the insulin dose at the time of exercise. Experience will dictate the amount of insulin to be taken, although guidelines do exist. If too much insulin is taken, the blood glucose will fall during exercise; if too little insulin is taken, performance will be reduced because of inability of the muscles to take up glucose.

Type 2 diabetes

In people with type 2 diabetes, a medical opinion should be sought before they undertake a major exercise programme. This group has a high prevalence of vascular disease. The medical practitioner would be wise to check blood pressure, give advice on drugs and diet, carry out an electrocardiogram as required, and give advice on appropriate exercise levels commensurate with fitness levels. That said, exercise in this group should be encouraged strongly within sensible limits.

Summary

Year on year, we continue to record an increase in prevalence of obesity in the developed world, developing countries showing equal enthusiasm for following suit. There is a worrying trend for this malaise to extend to children, and the overwhelming evidence indicates that this relates more to lack of exercise rather than to an increase in calorie intake. Associated with this is an increase in the incidence of type 2 diabetes, with projections indicating that this is likely to reach

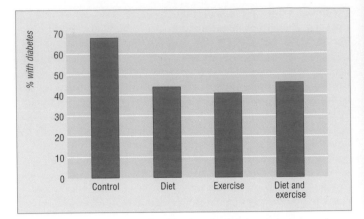

Progression to diabetes in the Da Qing impaired glucose tolerance and diabetes study. Adapted from Pan X, et al. *Diabetes Care* 1997;20:537-45

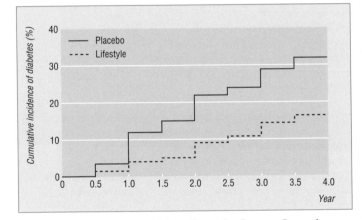

Progression to diabetes in the Diabetes Prevention Program Research Group. Adapted from Diabetes Prevention Program Research Group. *N Engl J Med* 2002;346:393-403

Guidelines for exercise in patients with diabetes treated with insulin

- Monitor blood glucose before, during (if possible), and after exercise
- Eat a snack of 15-40 g carbohydrate for every 30-60 minutes of exercise
- If on a twice daily insulin regimen, reduce intermediate acting insulin (isophane insulin) by 30% if exercise can be predicted and is likely to be strenuous
- Reduce pre-exercise short acting insulin by 30-50% according to experience
- Use non-exercising sites for insulin injection
- Monitor blood glucose for 24 hours after strenuous exercise

Guidelines for exercise in type 2 diabetes treated with diet or tablets

- Seek a medical opinion before undertaking an exercise programme; examination should include blood pressure, electrocardiogram, and assessment of glycaemic control
- Assess optimal exercise programme according to fitness level

epidemic proportions in the next 10 years. Solid epidemiological studies and randomised control studies have shown that exercise programmes can prevent the onset of diabetes, if not the onset of obesity. There is a growing database on interventions, including exercise programmes at home, school and in the workplace to counteract the increase in levels of obesity and diabetes, but those of us in a position to do so should encourage participation in exercise at whatever level.

1 Becque MD, Katch VL, Rocchini AP, Marks CR, Moorehead C. Coronary risk incidence of obese adolescents: reduction by exercise plus diet intervention. *Pediatrics* 1988;81:605

2 Health Development Agency. *Management of overweight and obesity.* London: Health Development Agency, 2003

3 Stampfer MJ, Malinow MR, Willett WC, Newcomer LM, Upson B, Ullmann D, et al. A prospective study of plasma homocyst(e)ine and risk of myocardial infarction in US physicians. *J Am Med Assoc* 1992;268:63-7

4 Helmrich SP, Ragland DR, Leung RW, Paffenbarger RS Jr. Physical activity and reduced occurrence of non-insulin-dependent diabetes mellitus. *N Engl J Med* 1991;325:147

19 Benefits of exercise in health and disease: challenges to implementing the evidence

John Buckley

The Department of Health in the United Kingdom, through its national service frameworks, has recommended that physical activity should play an important part in primary healthcare and secondary health care.

Physical activity, exercise, and sport

People who advise on or promote physical activity must acknowledge the patient's perceptions of physical activity. Failing to do so could result in setting inappropriate goals. A first step in preventing the client or patient being given inappropriate goals is for the health practitioner to clearly state what they mean by the terms physical activity, exercise, and sport. Comparison of these with what the client understands them to be clears the discussion of any misconceptions and misplaced advice.

Physical activity

Physical activity is considered to be any muscular movement above resting levels. It is an all encompassing concept that includes planned leisure pursuits (exercise and sport), as well as the physical movements needed for daily living. The prevalence of a number of illnesses or diseases is associated closely with people who expend <1500 kcal/week above their normal basal metabolic rate.

Declines in health that are related to inactivity (hypokinesis) and obesity are related more to the loss of physical activity in daily living as opposed to the debatable reduction in the populations' participation in organised exercise and sport. A look at the increased number of sports and fitness centres built in the United Kingdom in the last decade shows that certainly no decline has occurred in the people already engaged in organised sport and exercise. Reductions in energy expenditure within normal daily life, especially in non-sporty and non-exercising people, have increased greatly in the last two decades. This is a result of the increased attraction for sedentary leisure pursuits and decreases in the physicality of daily domestic-occupational tasks.

Chapter 18 described how physical inactivity (sloth) may be a larger contributor to the rise in obesity than dietary changes (gluttony) that have occurred in the past five decades. A weekly energy expenditure target of 1500 kcal can, depending on a person's initial state of health and fitness, at least prevent a decline if not improve physical and psychological well being. For the very sedentary, any activity is better than none, as this is the first stage in developing physical activity behaviour. The initial noticeable benefits are likely to be more psychological than physical. A sense of psychological well being from increased physical activity should be a primary concern, as this increases the chance of longer term adherence. If physical activity is not maintained, physical or psychological health gains become redundant.[1] Minimal activity (10 minutes) can improve acute states of enhanced well being for a number of hours to follow.

Exercise

Exercise typically is planned or structured physical activity that has an aim. The aim usually is to satisfy a physical,

---

Key challenges for medical and health practitioners in designing health based plans for physical activity

- Understanding the "dose" of physical activity (frequency, intensity, duration, and type) needed to achieve a health gain
- Psychosocial influences that act as barriers or avenues to people's participation

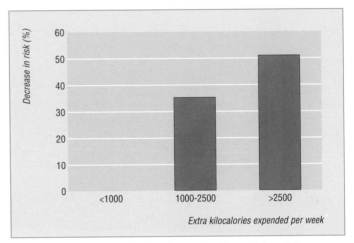

Energy expenditure and risk of cardiovascular disease. Adapted from Paffenbarger RS. *LifeFit*. Champaign, IL: Human Kinetics Publishers Inc, 1996

Causes of inactivity in daily life

- Increased use of cars
- Reduced use of pedestrian transport for short journeys
- Increased viewing of television
- Greater use of computers, electric domestic cleaning appliances and tools

---

Physical activity is best measured by the total energy expenditure involved in activity over the course of a day or week. From an epidemiological perspective, the recommended weekly energy expenditure target of 1500 kcal is most beneficial to sedentary people

---

Exercise was used traditionally as a means of preparing soldiers for battle, and since the industrial revolution, it has become prominent in improving sporting performance

psychological, or social need—typically a mixture of all three.

Sports performance targets provide natural motivation for maintaining exercise training. Motivation for regular participation is sometimes less easy to measure than athletic performance. Improving the social and enjoyment aspects of participation in health based exercise thus becomes an important aspect of any physical regimen. More frequent bouts (≥3 times a week) of more intense activity provide a training threshold at which physiological adaptation—better cardiorespiratory fitness, improved blood lipid profile and glucose control, and reduced insulin resistance—occurs. In such cases, people should breathe controllably harder for longer than 20-30 minutes. The activity can even be broken down into bouts as short as 10 minutes that total 30 minutes per day.

To acknowledge the overall psychological (cognitive and behavioural) milieu surrounding participation in physical activity is important. If the social environment of activity is enjoyable and promotes confidence and success, mental health and well being, and motivation, are more likely to increase.

Sport

Sport is simply physical activity within a competitive setting with rules. The intensity of activity usually is dictated externally by the competitive nature of the event. Although sport performance often is associated with physical prowess, for individual participants, the goals are in fact the potential psychological prizes. For individuals with illness or disease, sport usually is not an advisable arena for providing health promoting physical activity, because the physical risks easily can outweigh the benefits in many instances.

Fitness and health

Physical fitness is a composite of seven components that indicate the ability to perform a given task or physical activity. The benefits of improving fitness for health are twofold:

- Being able to sustain an active life to contribute functionally to personal needs or roles in family, community, and society
- Fitness is linked inversely with the incidence of morbidity of a variety of diseases and all cause mortality.

The seven components of fitness are the same for health or sport performance.

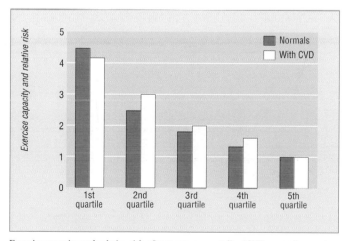

Exercise capacity and relative risk of premature mortality (CVD = cardiovascular disease). Adapted from Myers J et al. *New Engl J Med* 2002;346:793

Practical considerations

All physical activities need a combination, in varying degrees, of all seven components of fitness. Depending on the aim or purpose of the activity, one or a number of these seven

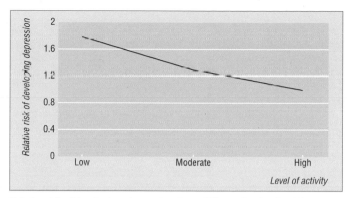

Relative risk of developing depression from different levels of activity. Adapted from Camacho TC et al. *Am J Epidemiol* 1991;134:220-31

Seven components of fitness

- Aerobic power*—described typically as VO_{2max}. This is the maximal amount of oxygen the body can take in and use. It is influenced by three factors: the lungs' ability to oxygenate the blood, the cardiovascular system's ability to deliver oxygenated blood to exercising muscles, and the muscles' ability to extract and use the oxygen to produce energy for sustained contractions. Inactivity or disease, or both, often impair one or several of these systems and so reduce a person's ability to function.
- Metabolic function from a health perspective relates to the ability to control blood sugar levels and from an exercise performance perspective the ability to deal with or buffer exercise related changes in muscle and blood pH. The latter shows that more active people also are able to tolerate and deal with higher levels of metabolites and prolong the time before muscular fatigue sets in.
- Muscular endurance relates to the anaerobic power of an individual and the ability to sustain the highest level of muscular contractions for periods between 30 seconds and two minutes. The older individual, whose life consists of short bouts of activity, is often limited more by a lack of strength and muscular endurance than by their aerobic fitness.
- Coordination, balance, and proprioception collectively describe a person's ability to perform a sequence of movements and their awareness of joint positions in space. For sports that involve dynamic skill (typically ball sports) and for the neurologically diseased (for example, those who have had a stroke or head injury or those with Parkinson's disease), this becomes the limiting factor in functional performance movement, regardless of strength, endurance, and flexibility.
- Aerobic endurance is the highest proportion of VO_{2max} at which a person can sustain (>20 minutes) activity. It is closely allied to the lactate threshold. Elite endurance athletes can sustain activity typically at >80% of their aerobic power, whereas sedentary or diseased people may be able to sustain activity at only 40-50% of their aerobic power. This means that inactive or diseased people not only have reduced capacities but cannot use as much of whatever capacity they possess compared with more active or fitter people.
- Flexibility is range of motion of a joint or group of joints. It is a function of the flexibility of the soft tissues in and around a joint (tendons, ligaments, and cartilage) plus the ability of the muscle's neurological unit to relax. All movement needs some flexibility. Regardless of the strength or endurance of an individual, flexibility can be a key limiting factor to function and performance.
- Muscular strength (power) is the absolute amount of power that can be generated for one maximal voluntary contraction. It is often represented by a one repetition maximum lift known as a "1-REP max". Muscular endurance—maintaining or increasing strength— is functionally advantageous to older people. Metabolic and cardiovascular benefits also are gained from increased muscular strength. A stronger muscle is a larger muscle, which needs more energy at rest and thus has an increased basal metabolic rate. This helps prevent accumulation of unhealthy adipose fat. The second benefit of stronger and larger muscles is that they have a greater volume of blood vessels. On exertion, a greater volume of blood vessels means a reduced rise in systolic blood pressure compared with a smaller muscle; the resultant workload on the heart is reduced.

*Aerobic is also known as cardiorespiratory

components becomes important.

For people who are pursuing cardiovascular health, aerobic power and endurance exercise typically are at the centre of such a fitness programme. In older people, however, quality of life in being able to independently operate in a domestic environment may be limited not by aerobic fitness but by their fitness to perform transient daily activities (getting out of a chair or opening a jar, climbing stairs, or short distance locomotion).

A direct relationship exists between a given activity and the rate of oxygen consumption of the body. Quantification of energy expenditure in this way is often described as a metabolic equivalent (MET). Activity above rest can be described as a multiple of this amount. Because an individual's maximal oxygen uptake can be estimated in a number of ways, METs can be used to estimate the potential cardiorespiratory challenge that a given activity may impose on a person. This is valuable when the intensity of activity, which may pose a risk for a person with cardiovascular disease, is evaluated.

Similarities between benefits of fitness training for athletes and patients

For highly trained athletes, small improvements in fitness may be the difference between winning and losing. For patients, small improvements may be the difference between a good or poor quality of independent life and a life with or free of symptoms (for example, angina, breathlessness, or muscle pain). Athletes will already have attained maximal capacity of the heart and lungs to deliver oxygen rich blood to the muscles; performance improvements are a result of subtle changes in muscle structure or biochemistry. This is similar for patients with heart or lung problems, because clinical pathology limits the amount of adaptable overload on the heart and lungs. Elite athletes and clinical patients thus must undertake training regimens (often interval or Fartlek type approaches) that improve the peripheral circulation and extraction and use of oxygen from skeletal muscle.

Monitoring health and exercise intensity that promotes fitness

Long established is that the frequency of activity needs to be more than twice a week for a health gain, whether for developing cardiorespiratory or muscular strength and endurance fitness. Activities that promote health need to be those that the person has some success and enjoyment from and that engage as many large muscle groups as possible (such as walking, running, swimming, cycling, or moderate intensity ball games). This leaves one important factor, the intensity of exercise. Different to all the other factors above, this needs most individual tailoring.

When laboratory based assessments of fitness are made, the recommendation is that less active people should be exercising at an intensity of 50-65% of their VO_{2max}. In real terms, a maximal test usually is not practical; however, heart rate or a person's rating of perceived exertion can be used to closely approximate a given percentage of VO_{2max}. An exercise intensity of 50-65% VO_{2max} can be approximated by one of the following methods:

- A heart rate of 65-80% of age estimated maximum (220—age)
- 50-65% maximum heart rate reserve, where the heart rate reserve is the difference between the resting and maximal heart rates
- Rating of perceived exertion on Borg's scale of 12 to 14 ("somewhat hard").[2]

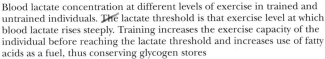

One MET is equivalent to the oxygen consumption of an individual at rest, where the rate of oxygen consumption (VO_2) is 3.5 ml/kg/min

Metabolic equivalents[*]

Physical activity	Metabolic equivalents
Hoovering	2.5-4
Mowing lawn (power mower on flat)	4.5-6
Walking 3miles per hour (5 km per hour)	4.5
Cycling 10 mile per hour (16 km per hour)	7.0
Jogging 7.5 miles per hour (12 km per hour at 8 minutes per mile)	12

[*]Data from ACSM guidelines for exercise testing and prescription. Boston: Lippincott, Williams and Wilkins, 2000 and Ainsworth BE et al. *Med Sci Sports Exerc* 1993;25:71

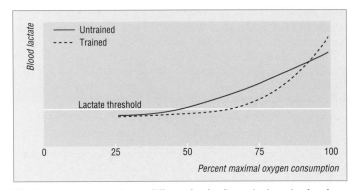

Blood lactate concentration at different levels of exercise in trained and untrained individuals. The lactate threshold is that exercise level at which blood lactate rises steeply. Training increases the exercise capacity of the individual before reaching the lactate threshold and increases use of fatty acids as a fuel, thus conserving glycogen stores

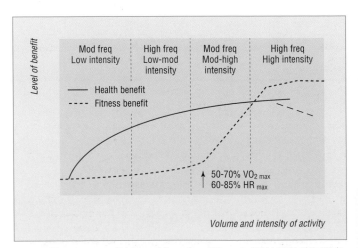

Activity "dose response." Adapted from Pate RR et al. *JAMA* 1996;273:402-7

As stated earlier, the threshold in people who train more regularly should be raised to a level in excess of 65% VO_{2max}, as demarcated by 75-90% maximal heart rate or 65-80% maximum heart rate reserve (independent of absolute aerobic performance). Interestingly, the rating of perceived exertion remains at the same value for this threshold in trained and untrained people.

Exercise prescription by heart rate

As a general rule, exercise should be prescribed at an intensity in the range of 40-85% of functional capacity. For normal subjects, this is usually between 60% and 80% of functional capacity. In groups that are at risk, this is reduced to 40-60% in the first instance.

Heart rate reserve is calculated by subtracting the resting heart rate from the maximum heart rate. The product of the exercise intensity as a percentage and the heart rate reserve is added to the resting heart rate to obtain the training range of heart rate that is needed—for example,

Maximum heart rate 160 beats per minute
Resting heart rate 70 beats per minute
Heart rate reserve 90 beats per minute
40% functional capacity = $(0.4 \times 90) + 70$ = 106 beats per minute
80% functional capacity = $(0.8 \times 90) + 70$ = 142 beats per minute

Fitness and cardiovascular disease

High cholesterol and hypertension are two of the main causes of cardiovascular disease. These risk factors are modified by physical activity; however, inactivity and especially low cardiorespiratory fitness are both independent risk factors that possess equivalent if not greater potency than these two key risk factors. This is not widely acknowledged yet. A proposed key mechanism, by which exercise training reduces the chances of ischaemia, is the improved coronary blood flow on exertion.[3]

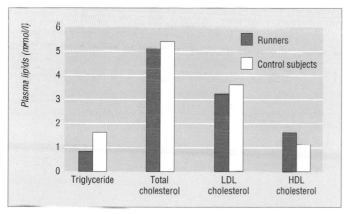

Comparison in lipid levels in men who run regularly and control subjects. Similar effects were seen in women subjects (LDL = low density lipoprotein; HDL = high density lipoprotein). Adapted from Wood PD, Haskell WH. *Lipids* 1979;14:417

Risks of participation

The physical risk of injury or illness is often given as a reason for non-participation.[4] Absolute (acute) and relative risk (chronic development or reduction of illness or injury) have been identified. For cardiac patients, participation in rehabilitative exercise results in a relative risk reduction of 25-30% in premature all cause mortality.[5] The absolute risk of a cardiac event leading to mortality from physical exertion has been described in a number of different ways.[6] In an individual without known coronary heart disease, the risk of an event is about one in 1.5 million. For cardiac populations involved in

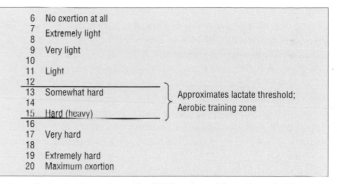

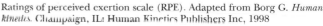

Ratings of perceived exertion scale (RPE). Adapted from Borg G. *Human kinetics.* Champaign, IL: Human Kinetics Publishers Inc, 1998

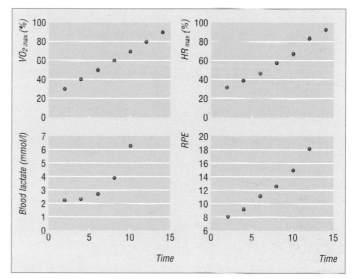

Relationship between lactate threshold (bottom left) and percentage VO_{2max} (top left), % HR_{max} (top right), and ratings of perceived exertion (RPE) (bottom right)

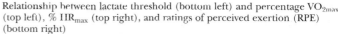

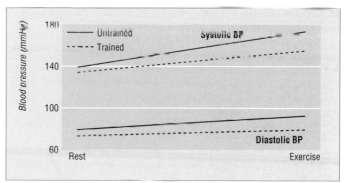

Blood pressure levels at rest and during exercise before and after short courses of fitness training. Adapted from Clausen JP et al. *Circulation* 1969;40:143

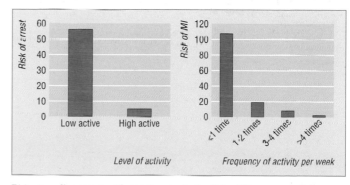

Risk of cardiac events with regular physical activity (MI = myocardial infarction). Adapted from Siscovick DS et al. *New Engl J Med* 1984;311:874-7 and Mittleman MA et al. *New Engl J Med* 1993;329:1677-83

rehabilitative exercise, Froelicher and Myers summarised numerous studies reporting the incident of events.[6] More than 80% of exertion related events were cardiac arrests compared with <20% myocardial infarctions. The largest study reported an incidence of 8.9 events per million patient hours, with 86% being successfully resuscitated; thus, the death rate was very low at 1.3 per million patient hours. The above statistics clearly show the low risk of appropriately designed exercise training and the value of having defibrillation equipment and trained personnel leading exercise in those at risk of a cardiac event.

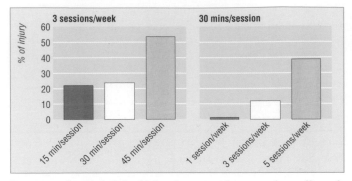

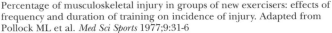

Percentage of musculoskeletal injury in groups of new exercisers: effects of frequency and duration of training on incidence of injury. Adapted from Pollock ML et al. *Med Sci Sports* 1977;9:31-6

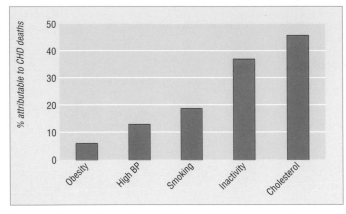

Potency of coronary heart disease risk factors (CHD = coronary heart disease; BP = blood pressure). Adapted from Britton A, McPherson K. National Heart Forum 2000, British Heart Foundation

Of interest

Health practitioners who are regularly physically active themselves are three to four times better at persuading patients to become active compared with their sedentary counterparts.[7] Only about 12% of general practitioners know that inactivity is the second most potent risk factor for coronary heart disease after high lipid levels.

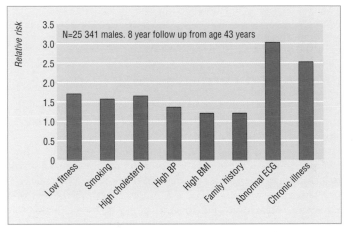

Adjusted relative risks of cardiovascular disease for eight predictors (BMI = body mass index; BP = blood pressure; ECG = electrocardiogram). Data from Farrell SW et al. *Med Sci Sports Exerc* 1998;30:899 and Blair SN et al. *JAMA* 1996;276:205

1 Biddle S, Mutrie N. *Psychology of physical activity; determinants, well-being and interventions*. London: Routledge, 2001
2 Borg G. *Borg's rating of perceived exertion and pain scales*. Champaign, IL: Human Kinetics, 1998
3 Hambrecht R, Adams V, Erbs S, Linke A, Krankel N, Shu Y, et al. Regular physical activity improves endothelial function in patients with coronary artery disease by increasing phosphorylation of endothelial nitric oxide synthase. *Circulation* 2003;107:3152-8
4 Dishman R, ed. *Advances in exercise adherence*. Champaign, IL: Human Kinetics, 1994
5 Jolliffe JA, Rees K, Taylor RS, Thompson D, Oldridge N, Ebrahim S, et al. Exercise-based rehabilitation for coronary heart disease. *Cochrane Data Base Syst Rev* 2003:CD001800
6 Froelicher VF, Myers J. *Exercise and the heart*, 4th ed. Philadelphia: WB Saunders, 2000
7 McKenna J, Naylor PJ, McDowell N. Barriers to physical activity promotion by general practitioners and practice nurses. *Br J Sports Med* 1998;32:242-7

Further reading

- Astrand P-O, Rodahl K. *Textbook of work physiology; physiological bases of exercise*. Champaign, IL: Human Kinetics, 2003
- British Heart Foundation. (www.bhf.org.uk)
- Buckley J, Holmes J, Mapp G. *Exercise on prescription; cardiovascular activity for health*. Oxford: Butterworth Heinemann, 1999
- Pollock ML, Franklin BA, Balady GJ, Chaitman BL, Fleg JL, Fletcher B, et al. Resistance exercise in individuals with and without cardiovascular disease: benefits, rationale, safety and prescription: an advisory from the committee on Exercise, Rehabilitation, and Prevention. *Circulation* 2000;101:828-33
- Thompson PD, Buchner D, Pina IL, Balady GJ, Williams MA, Marcus BH, et al. Exercise and physical activity in the prevention and treatment of atherosclerotic cardiovascular disease. *Circulation* 2003;107:3109-16

20   Active in later life

Archie Young, Susie Dinan

Regular physical activity brings important health benefits at any age. Its importance for health in old age is highlighted repeatedly in the English national service framework for older people. Any potential hazards can be reduced by education and guidance of participants.

Prevention of disease

Regular physical activity helps prevent conditions important in "old age," notably osteoporosis, non-insulin dependent diabetes mellitus, hypertension, ischaemic heart disease, stroke, and perhaps some cancers, specifically colon cancer.

Prevention of disability

Not only does regular physical activity play an important part in preventing disease, its function preserving effects are also important. Appropriate physical training improves the functional abilities of people with disabling symptoms of intermittent claudication, angina pectoris, heart failure, asthma, and chronic bronchitis. Frail elderly patients with multiple disabilities may also derive functional benefits from graded physical training.

Even healthy elderly people lose strength at a rate of some 1-2% per year and power at a rate of some 3-4% per year. In addition, many elderly people have further problems because of the presence of chronic disease. The resulting weakness has important functional consequences for the performance of everyday activities. In the English National Fitness Survey, nearly half of women and 15% of men aged 70-74 years had a power to weight ratio (for extension of the lower limb) too low to be confident of being able to mount a 30 cm step without a hand rail. A similar argument applies for endurance capacity: 80% of women and 35% of men aged 70-74 years had an aerobic power to weight ratio so low that they would be unable to sustain comfortably a walk at 3 miles an hour. Similarly, at least a third of women and nearly a quarter of men aged 70-74 years had shoulder abduction so restricted that they would be unable to wash their hair without difficulty.

Regular exercise increases strength, endurance, and flexibility. In percentage terms, the improvements seen in elderly people are similar to those in younger people. Supervised programmes of specific exercises to improve strength and dynamic balance have been shown to be effective in reducing falls. International clinical guidelines now include exercise as an important component of an effective multifactorial intervention for the prevention of falls.

Prevention of immobility

For those who are severely disabled, immobility has substantial hazards. Movement, even in the absence of a training effect, contributes to the prevention of faecal impaction, deep vein thrombosis, and gravitational oedema.

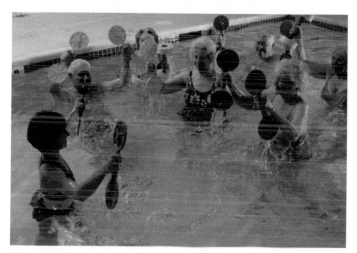

Elderly people taking part in a water exercise class

Physical activity helps prevent

- Disease—osteoporosis, non-insulin dependent diabetes, hypertension, ischaemic heart disease, stroke, anxiety, depression, colonic cancer?
- Disability—caused by intermittent claudication, angina pectoris, heart failure, asthma, chronic bronchitis, age related weakness
- Problems—arthritic pain, poor sleep, falls, fractures
- Immobility—can cause faecal impaction, deep vein thrombosis, gravitational oedema
- Isolation—can cause loneliness or depression or both

Strength = the ability to exert force

Power = force × speed

Improvements produced by exercise

In two studies by the Royal Free Hospital:

- Women aged 75-93 years increased their strength by 24-30% with just 12 weeks of strength training (equivalent to a "rejuvenation" of strength by 15-20 years)
- Women aged 80-93 years produced a 15% mean increase in their aerobic power to weight ratio with 24 weeks of endurance training (equivalent to a "rejuvenation" of endurance of 15 years)

Prevention of isolation

In addition to its physiological effects, recreational exercise offers important opportunities for socialisation. It also permits the emotional benefits of socially acceptable touching, unconnected with dependence and the need for personal care, a rarity for many long bereaved elderly people.

Providing guidance and opportunity

What type of activity?

Any exercise programme to improve general fitness must include activities to develop strength, endurance, flexibility, and coordination in a progressive and enjoyable way. It must use all major muscle groups in exercises that train through each individual's fullest possible pain free ranges of movement. An exercise programme for older people must also aim to load the bones; target major functional, postural, and pelvic floor muscles; include practice of functional movements; and emphasise the development of body awareness and balance skills. A combination of regular recreational walking and swimming (both at an intensity that is comfortably challenging), preferably combined with specific exercises to improve strength and flexibility, will meet most of these criteria for most people. Many older people also welcome the opportunity to participate in group exercise.

How much is enough?

Until recently, published guidelines recommended vigorous physical activity to achieve the expected health benefits. Ample evidence now shows that substantial health benefits can be obtained by an approach that is more temperate and, arguably, more likely to be sustained. For endurance activities such as walking and swimming, this approach is based on five episodes of 30 minutes a week of exercise at a moderate intensity—that is with an effort that makes the participant feel "comfortably challenged," warm, and breathing a little more heavily. (Of course, the speed of walking that is "comfortably challenging" will vary considerably from person to person.)

The older and frailer the participant, the greater the potential benefit from the inclusion of strengthening, stretching, balance, and coordination activities and the greater the need for individually tailored exercise guidance from a suitably trained specialist (see below).

Exercise groups

A short chapter cannot teach how a seniors' exercise group should be run. Rather, we offer guidance to health professionals on areas to consider when they assess an exercise group to which they might refer patients or when they seek specialist training to allow them to lead groups safely and successfully.

All sessions should start and finish gradually with a warm up and warm down. For frailer participants, many of the activities should be related closely to life and maintaining independence. Techniques of lifting, walking, transferring (moving from sitting to standing, standing to lying), and even crawling should be specifically taught and discussed. Information about the specific benefits of particular exercises is greatly appreciated—for example, shoulder mobility for reaching zips; stamina for "energy" and less breathlessness during exertion; or quadriceps, handgrip, and biceps strengthening for carrying shopping or using the bus.

Above all, fitness must be fun. Important factors can be variety, the use of appropriate equipment, games, music, and opportunities for socialising (but beware of ageist assumptions about what is appropriate).

Programming

The aim is a long term commitment to a mixture of evidence based activities. The combinations should be tailored to the individual's health, fitness, functional ability, tastes, interests, and means. A home exercise programme can usefully complement the organised sessions. Provision must be made for a wide range of initial levels of habitual physical activity and for a variety of disabilities.

Guidance on physical activity at any age

- 30 minutes of moderate intensity physical activity on at least five days of the week will improve health
- Two 15 minute periods of moderate activity in a day can be beneficial and a good way to start
- Every little counts towards the 30 minutes' activity total. To start with, if 15 minutes sounds too much, take a "little and often" approach, advising the participant to progress steadily from just three minutes until three minutes becomes five minutes, then five minutes twice a day, increasing to 10, 15, and finally 30 minutes of moderate activity
- Maximum benefit to health probably will be gained with 20 minutes of vigorous endurance activity three times a week, 20 minutes of strengthening activity twice a week plus daily stretching, balance, and coordination activities
- Any activity is better than none, and even once a week is better than nothing
- It is never too late to start
- It is best to select enjoyable activities

Implications for teachers when running "fitness for seniors" classes

- Emphasise posture and technique
- Give more teaching points and repeat more often
- Give more warning of directional and step changes
- Improve own body language and demonstration skills
- Improve own observation, monitoring, and correction skills
- Offer more choices
- Offer more information
- Be polished and punctual

A warm up lubricates joints, warms muscles, rehearses skills, and gradually increases demand on the heart and lungs

A warm down consists principally of slow rhythmic exercises to preserve venous return as muscle and skin vasodilation gradually return to resting levels. It may also incorporate relaxation, held stretches, additional strengthening, and falls management activities in sitting or lying positions

Exercises might include walking, swimming, weight training, circuit training, step training, exercise to music, dancing, chair work, tai chi, tennis, and bowls

Programmes should provide opportunities for exclusive seniors' sessions and integration with other age groups for selected activities. Opportunities to socialise should be scheduled at all activities. Year round programming is essential. Off peak timing improves use of resources but must not exclude the many older people still in employment. Teachers should be professionally registered with specialist qualifications (see section on education and training) and must be paid accordingly, but concessionary rates and discretionary financial assistance may be considered for individual participants.

Participants must be involved in planning, selecting, and evaluating the programme. The setting should be friendly to older people in terms of public transport, parking, access, ambience, ventilation, lighting, refreshments, floor surfaces, and changing and toilet facilities. Thought should be given for those with a disability (for example, stair rails, large print notices, and wheelchair access). Promotional material should feature appropriate older role models.

Safety

Injury prevention is a high priority. Even stiffness and minor overuse injuries reduce enjoyment and adherence and can often be avoided. An adequate warm up, the selection of safe exercises and movement patterns, regular monitoring of body alignment and exercise intensity, and an appropriate warm down are important. Precise, audible teaching instructions and visible skilled demonstrations are essential. Skilful class management and observation are needed to ensure safety in seniors' fitness sessions. These issues are taught in specialist courses for health and exercise professionals who are training to run exercise groups for older people.

Opinion is divided over the place of informed consent forms and medical release forms for older adults embarking on unaccustomed physical activity. On the one hand, everything possible to minimise any potential hazard needs to be done, and it seems likely that medical review will contribute usefully. On the other hand, legitimate concerns exist about overmedicalisation of recreational activities and the impossibility of detecting all potentially important pathologies. Furthermore, medical review has tended to ensure "safety" by exclusion, failing to recognise that those people identified as carrying a higher risk of adverse events during physical activity (for example, a hypertensive person with diabetes) are the very ones who stand to gain most by participation. Fortunately, things are changing, and the need is recognised for an "enabling," pre-exercise medical review that will facilitate safe and effective recreational participation by all older people.

What, then, should doctors do, especially as they will usually be less able than the specialist exercise teacher to advise on the individualised prescription of particular exercises or activities? The doctor has three responsibilities:

- To identify pathologies that are present and ensure they and all drugs are communicated accurately to the exercise teacher
- To highlight any ways they consider the safe conduct of exercise might be influenced by the:
  — diagnoses (for example, susceptibility to angina, shortness of breath, arrhythmias, joint pain, and confusion)
  — drugs (for example, by suppressing pain, producing a bradycardia unrepresentative of exercise intensity, or increasing susceptibility to postural hypotension)
- To educate the person exercising to recognise early symptoms that might indicate the exercise programme is, in some way, unsuitable for them and their particular chronic pathologies. Patients with osteoarthritic knees should be taught to recognise and respect an increase in pain, stiffness, or swelling

Implications for planning when running "fitness for seniors" classes

- Include seniors
  in planning and staffing
  in evaluation
  in promotional material
- Pre-exercise review of health information and functional needs
- First session is an individual assessment
- The evidence base
- Individualised or tailored programmes
- Progressive and multilevel programmes
- Mixture of activities
- Ensure essential facilities
- Appropriate scheduling and costing
- Include socialisation time
- Include educational opportunities

Competence to run such fitness groups for seniors implies theoretical knowledge and practical experience in selecting and supervising safe, appropriate exercises according to the participants' particular medical problems, such as unsteadiness, breathlessness, angina, arthritis, osteoporosis, or inability to stand

Extract from an exercise referral form used by health professionals to transfer clinical information meaningfully to the exercise practitioner. (Adapted from Dinan, Young, Iliffe, Wallace, unpublished)

The patient with a history of mild, controlled heart failure should be taught that increased breathing during exercise is normal but that a decrease in the level of exercise required to provoke shortness of breath is abnormal.

Thus, clinical responsibility rests with the referrer. On the other hand, responsibility for the administration, design, and delivery of the programme rests with the leisure management and instructor team or the exercise practitioner service, or both. To take this share of the overall responsibility, those supervising the conduct of the exercise must be able to demonstrate appropriate training and continuing professional development.

Education and training

In many respects, an elderly person is like an athlete: both often perform near their limits. The instructing and supervising skills needed to ensure optimal performance and safety are important and specialised.

In England, the Register of Exercise Professionals operates a national competency based registration process. Registered teachers, trainers, and instructors are properly qualified, insured, and work to a code of ethical practice. (Somewhat similar registration schemes are run by Fitness Scotland, Fitness Wales and Fitness Northern Ireland.) Health professionals can identify suitably qualified exercise professionals with the help of a free database search facility operated by the Register of Exercise Professionals.

The qualification requirements of exercise and fitness teachers in the United Kingdom are undergoing considerable change. The National Occupational Standards describe the knowledge base and practical competencies that exercise and fitness teachers must possess. The teaching of exercise and fitness to older adults—a "special population group"—is sited at level 3 and is one of the more advanced qualifications. At this level, requirements include the ability to develop long term physical activity programmes adapted to accommodate the heterogeneity and physical limitations of older people. This needs knowledge of the ways in which ageing and medical conditions may affect exercise performance and participation. The new level 3 national occupation standards and qualifications now apply as from the middle of 2004. Currently, those teaching this age group can obtain exercise and fitness qualifications through courses certified by the qualifications of the central YMCA, and exercise and movement qualifications through Extend, Excel 2000, and the Keep Fit Association. From the middle of 2004, all training providers working in this specialist field will need to align their education and training to the revised level 3 National Occupational Standards. Training at Level 4 is currently under development. It will include specialist exercise certification for exercise and health professionals working with medium-to-high risk patient groups, including frailer older people.

Summary

Physical activity is an important therapeutic and preventive option for middle aged and older patients. Health professionals are well placed to endorse the "use it or lose it" message and to give the advice and authoritative encouragement an older person may need to begin or return to physical recreation. We welcome the growth of exercise referral schemes and urge other health professionals in primary and secondary care to develop close working partnerships with exercise professionals and the management and providers of local recreational facilities. Such schemes are popular with primary care professionals, service commissioners, leisure centre managers, instructors, and

ACTIVITY PLAN ACKNOWLEDGEMENT

If you are *satisfied* with Patient Activity Plan, please tick box below, sign and file.

If you are *not satisfied* please tick box below left, sign and return by Post or Fax, or telephone 5 working days prior to the proposed start date.

By completing the Activity Plan Acknowledgement form you are not assuming responsibility for the administration or delivery of the exercise programme.

The exercise programme will be administered by qualified staff all of whom have specialist training in working with special populations. The premises meet all health and safety criteria and are the responsibility of the management.

- Clinical responsibility rests with the referrer.
- Responsibility for the exercise assessment and the administration, design and delivery of the programme rests with the leisure management instructor team and/or exercise practitioner service.
- Responsibility for consenting to take part in the exercise programme, observing the advised precautions and following the plan and the exercise practitioners guidance rests with the participant where possible.

I am satisfied with this patient's Activity Plan
I need to discuss this patient's Activity Plan further

Referring Clinician's signature _____   Date: _____
Tel no: _____   Fax no: _____

Form used by the referring doctor to acknowledge receipt of the exercise practitioner's proposals for an individual patient's activity plan. (Adapted from Dinan, Young, Iliffe, Wallace, unpublished)

Agencies

- Age Concern England: Astral House, 1268 London Road, Norbury, London SW16 4ER (tel: 020 8765 7200; email: ace@ace.org.uk; website: www.ageconcern.org.uk)
- Age Concern Scotland: 113 Rose Street, Edinburgh EH2 3DT (tel: 0131 220 3345; email: enquiries@acscot.org.uk; website: www.ageconcernscotland.org.uk)
- Age Concern Wales: 4th Floor, 1 Cathedral Road, Cardiff CF11 9SD (tel: 029 2037 1566; email: enquiries@accymru.org.uk; website: www.accymru.org.uk)
- Age Concern Northern Ireland: 3 Lower Crescent, Belfast BT7 1NR (tel: 0289 024 5729; email: info@ageconcernni.org; website: www.ageconcernni.org)
- Association of Retired and Persons over 50: Windsor House, 1270 London Road, London SW16 4DH (tel: 0208 764 3344; email: info@arp050.org.uk; website: www.arp050.org.uk)
- Help the Aged: 207-221 Pentonville Road, London N1 9UZ (tel: 020 7278 1114; email: info@helptheaged.org.uk; website: www.helptheaged.org.uk)
- Ramblers Association: 2nd Floor, Camelford House, 87-90 Albert Embankment, London SE1 7TW (tel: 020 7339 8500; email: ramblers@london.ramblers.org.uk; website: www.ramblers.org.uk)

Training organisations

- YMCA Fitness Industry Training: 111 Great Russell Street, London WC1B 3NP (tel: 0207 343 1850; email: info@ymcafit.org.uk; website: www.ymcafit.org.uk)
- Extend: 2 Place Farm, Wheathampstead, Herts AL4 8SB (tel: 01582 832760; email: admin@extend.org.uk; website: www.extend.org.uk)
- Excel 2000: 1a North Street, Sheringham, Norfolk NR26 8LW (tel: 01263 825 670; email: excel2000@lineone.net)
- Later Life Training: 44 Egerton Gardens, London W13 8HQ (email: info@laterlifetraining.co.uk; website: www.laterlifetraining.co.uk)
- British Heart Foundation National Centre for Physical Activity and Health: Loughborough University, Leics LE11 3TU (tel: 01509 223 259; email: bhfactive@lists.lboro.ac.uk; website: www.bhfactive.org.uk)

Senior friendly multipurpose fitness equipment

- Davies Sports: Excelsior House, Ashby Park, Ashby de la Zouche, Leicestershire LE65 1NG (tel: 0845 120 4515; email: enquiries@daviessports.co.uk; website: www.daviessports.co.uk)
- Powersport International Ltd: Queen's Road, Bridgend Industrial Estate, Bridgend, South Wales CF31 3UT (tel: 01656 678 910; email: info@powersport-int.com; website: www.powersport-int.co.uk)

patients. Their continuing growth will now be supported by national policy guidelines for quality assurance that have been developed in response to a commission from the Department of Health. Finally, do remember that if you set your own example as an active person, you will have a positive impact on your patients' behaviour.

The photograph of the water exercise class is with permission of Sean O'Brien, Custom Medical Stock Photo/Science Photo Library. We thank Cliff Collins for his help in describing the Register of Exercise Professionals and the current structure of training and certification. We also thank our collaborators Steve Iliffe and Paul Wallace for permission to include the forms on pages 99 and 100. Susie Dinan is a Director of Later Life Training Ltd, a company that aims to provide specialist, safe and effective exercise training for professionals working with vulnerable older people (for example, Falls Prevention) and accessible information to older people and their carers to help them increase participation in physical activity and tailored exercise.

National governing bodies

- Register of Exercise Professionals: 3rd Floor, 8-10 Crown Hill, Croydon, Surrey CR0 1RZ (tel: 020 8686 6464; email: info@exerciseregister.org; website: www.exerciseregister.org)
- Fitness Scotland: 2 Lint Riggs, Falkirk FK1 1DG (tel: 01324 886 506; email: office@fitness-scotland.com; website: www.fitness-scotland.com)
- Fitness Wales: 1b Clarke Street, Ely Bridge, Cardiff CF5 5AL (tel: 029 20 57 5155; email: enquiries@fitnesswales.co.uk; website: www.fitnesswales.co.uk)
- Fitness Northern Ireland: The Robinson Centre, Montgomery Road, Belfast BT6 9JD (tel: 0289 070 4080; email: fitnessni@aol.com)

Sports councils

- Sport England: 3rd Floor, Victoria House, Bloomsbury Square, London WC1B 4SE (tel: 0207 273 1500; email: info@sportengland.org; website: www.sportengland.org)
- Sport Scotland: Caledonia House, South Gyle, Edinburgh EH12 9DQ (tel: 0131 317 7200; email: library@sportscotland.org.uk; website: www.sportscotland.org.uk)
- Sports Council for Wales: Sophia Gardens, Cardiff CF11 9SW (tel: 029 2030 0500; email: publicity@scw.co.uk; website: www.sports-council-wales.co.uk)
- Sports Council for Northern Ireland: House of Sport, Upper Malone Road, Belfast BT9 5LA (tel: 028 90 381 222; email: info@sportni.net; website: www.sportni.net)

National occupational standards awarding bodies

- NVQ: Head Office, Edexcel, One90 High Holborn, London WC1V 7BH (tel: 0870 240 9800; website: www.cdexcel.org.uk)
- City and Guilds: 1 Giltspur Street, London EC1A 9DD (tel: 0207 294 2800; email: enquiry@city-and-guilds.co.uk; website: www.city-and-guilds.co.uk)
- OCR Examinations: Regional Office South East, Veritas House, 125 Finsbury Pavement, London EC2A 1NQ (tel: 020 7256 7819; email: ocr-south-east@ocr.org.uk; website: www.ocr.org.uk)
- Central YMCA Qualifications: 112 Great Russell Street, London WC1B 3NP (tel: 020 7343 1800; email: info@cyq.org.uk; website: www.cyq.org.uk)
- SQA: Hanover House, 24 Douglas Street, Glasgow G2 7NP (tel: 0845 279 1000; email: customer@sqa.org.uk; website: www.sqa.org.uk)
- SkillsActive: Castlewood House, 77-91 New Oxford Street, London WC1A 1PX (tel: 020 7632 2000; email: skills@skillsactive.com; website: www.skillsactive.org.uk)

21 Physiotherapy, sports injuries, and reacquisition of fitness

Caryl Becker, Lynn Booth

Chartered physiotherapists' management of sports injuries is a continuum of stages. Chartered physiotherapists also are involved in injury prevention and performance enhancement, including musculoskeletal profiling, coach and athlete education, and specific conditioning programmes.

Sports injury management

Chartered physiotherapists working with sportspeople face the challenge of trying to return an injured athlete to training and competition in as short a time as possible, while making sure that reinjury does not occur.

Athletes continually push their boundaries and tend to expect nothing less from their medical and support team. Successful treatment of injury is best achieved by good cooperation, commitment and communication. A team approach must be the priority when dealing with injured athletes, who should be seen as a whole and not solely as an injury. Athletes want to return to competition not just fitness.

Assessment and diagnosis

The first priority of physiotherapists treating an injury is a full and detailed subjective and objective assessment. Only after a thorough evaluation can a diagnosis be made and an appropriate treatment programme established.

Sports injuries can involve several structures; although some are severe enough to result in hospitalisation, most are usually soft tissue injuries that involve the muscle, ligament, or tendon. These injuries can be divided into grade 1, 2, or 3 injuries. The severity of injury will determine the type of treatment needed.[1]

Treatment

From the physiotherapist's viewpoint, the parameters of fitness can be classified broadly into five areas. Chartered physiotherapists continually work towards attaining full fitness. Treatment depends on the stage of the healing (inflammatory) process and will be instigated and modified depending on the athlete's signs and symptoms.

Immediate treatment

In acute injuries, the first aim of treatment is to reduce pain, inflammation, and swelling. Whatever the method used, the emphasis is on creating the best environment in which healing can take place. Initial treatment often takes place at the training venue or competition site, with the doctor, physiotherapist, or first aider being the first port of call. All medical personnel who find themselves in this position should hold a valid and up to date first aid certificate. Sports doctors and physiotherapists are encouraged to hold an acute trauma certificate: for example, the Association of Chartered Physiotherapists in Sports Medicine's advanced trauma life support course.

Mobility

Mobility can be achieved by increasing the range of movement in a joint, lengthening a shortened muscle, and releasing the tension on the neural system.

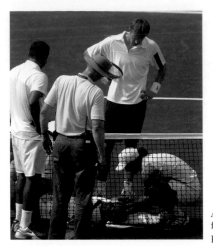

Athletes require a great deal from their medical team. With permission from Getty Images

---

Aims of physiotherapy treatment

To decrease
- Pain
- Inflammation
- Swelling

To increase
- Joint range of movement
- Muscle strength
- Muscle length

Stages in physiotherapists' management of sport injuries

- Assessment
- Diagnosis
- Treatment
- Functional rehabilitation
- Fitness testing

Joint consultation between the sports physician; physiotherapist; other relevant sport science, sports medicine, and coaching staff; and the athlete is preferential when identifying goals and objectives of treatment. This offers the athlete awareness of the targets being set for recovery

---

Fitness parameters

- Flexibility
- Endurance
- Strength
- Speed
- Skill

Treatment to reduce pain, inflammation, and swelling

First 72 hours	After first 72 hours
● Protection	● Massage
● Rest	● Electrotherapy
● Ice	● Acupuncture
● Compression	● Deep tissue work
● Elevation	

Range of movement

Mobilisations and manipulations can increase range of movement of joints.[2] These movements need to be physiological and accessory in nature in order to be sure that a joint has fully regained range. At times, the range of movement may be limited by protective muscle spasm or the presence of trigger points in the muscles. A physiotherapist would release the spasm and trigger points by using massage, acupuncture, and other deep soft tissue work.

Stretching

Stretching is one of the most widely debated principles, with much contradiction evident in the research. Stretching was shown to relax stiff tight muscles and can be static or dynamic in nature.[4] Static stretches may improve range of motion, are traditionally held for 15-30 seconds, and are performed lightly to the point of discomfort (not into pain). Shrier and Gossal believe static stretching reduces viscoelasticity and increases stretch tolerance.[3] They also suggest that patients stretch until they feel a certain amount of tension but no pain. As the stretch is held, stress relaxation occurs and the muscle's force decreases. When less tension is felt, because of changes in viscoelasticity and analgesic effect, the muscle length can again be increased until the original tension is felt. A muscle increased in length always should be strengthened in this new range to avoid injury.

Another method of increasing muscle length is proprioceptive neuromuscular facilitation—this allows for a complex movement to be strengthened and lengthened rather than an isolated muscle.[5] Patterns of proprioceptive neuromuscular facilitation are more functional in nature and help improve joint awareness, strength, and neuromuscular control.[6] Techniques for proprioceptive neuromuscular facilitation, such as hold and relax, aid muscle lengthening and are useful when faced with a shortened muscle that the athlete is finding difficult to relax. It is based on the concept that maximum relaxation follows maximum contraction, therefore allowing a greater stretch.

The optimal duration and frequency of stretching may vary between muscle groups and individuals, which emphasises the importance of programmes being specific and individualised. The athlete, more than anyone, is best placed to find out what length, frequency, and type of stretching they respond to best.

Neural tension

Mobilising neural structures may be required when adverse neural tension is present. Adverse neural tension may be the cause of pain, reduced range of movement, and decreased function. Common nerve stretches would be the "slump" for the lumbar nerves and upper limb tension tests for the upper arm and neck. These stretches can be given to the athlete as a form of treatment as well as a home exercise programme. Mobilisation of the thoracic spine when the patient sits with their legs straight out in front of them helps stretch parasympathetic nerves, which can influence tension on the neuromuscular system.

Functional rehabilitation

Regaining function is the main focus of all treatment, with inadequate rehabilitation being a major cause of reinjury. A common mistake many physiotherapists make is to rehabilitate an athlete without making sure that the regimen is specific enough to the individual sport.

Stretching

- Stretching remains popular with athletes, as many believe it prevents injuries, but the evidence for this is limited
- Warm up not stretching prevents injury
- If injury prevention is the primary objective and the range of movement needed for the activity is not extreme, athletes should stop stretching before exercise and increase the warm up aspect of preparation for competition[3]

Dynamic stretching

- Dynamic stretching involves rhythmic movement through available range of movement and prepares the musculature for the ballistic motion in all sports
- Seen as an important element to the warm up process, it should precede static stretching, as an active warm up before stretching has been shown to result in a greater improvement in range of movement than warm up without stretching

---

> When a physiotherapist prescribes stretching, they must explain to the athlete why it is being done, what outcome is being sought, and what structures are being affected

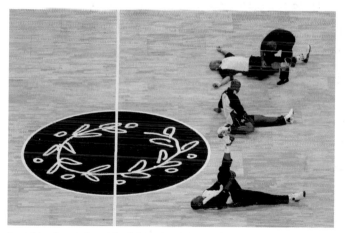

Stretching is popular with athletes, but it is a widely debated principle. Reproduced with permission from Getty Images

---

Factors in rehabilitation

- Stabilisation
- Speed
- Strength
- Power
- Endurance
- Skill

Stabilisation

Core stability provides the trunk with the support it needs to allow forces from the arms and legs to be efficient, strong, and effective when generating power. The stabilising muscles of the pelvic and shoulder girdles need to be trained specifically to perform the task of "holding" rather than "moving."[7]

Stabilisation exercises should be progressive in nature and include working on a gym ball and using resistance bands or tubing and medicine balls. When this equipment is used, the exercises should remain sport specific, interesting, and fun. Break down of a sports specific action or technique to manageable sections is one of the ways that physiotherapists can replicate what happens in training or competition and in the treatment room or gym. Each aspect of the skill is brought together to perform the task needed for that particular sport.

At the end of treatment, physiotherapists should be able to say, with confidence, that an athlete is able to stabilise (as opposed to bracing, which is the use of the global mobilisers rather than the local stabilisers[8]) in a functional way, while performing activities related to their sport.

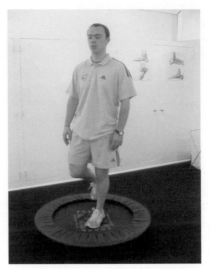

Stabilisation activity that introduces a sport specific element while balancing on a mini trampoline

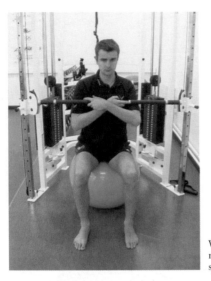

Working core stabilisers in a more functional position for a sport such as canoeing

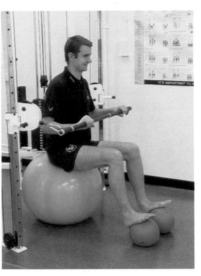

Progression of activity by reducing stability of lower limbs

Improved stabilisation

Lowers
- Risk of injury
- Compensatory movements of trunk

Raises
- Efficiency of muscle power
- Control of body motion and momentum
- Capacity to generate speed
- Balance and coordination
- Posture

Core stability exercises should never be seen as the panacea for all lower back pain, but an understanding of their importance and relevance to athletes is vital

Speed

Speed in forwards, backwards, and lateral directions is important in many sports and each has to be worked on specifically. By adding in stops, starts, and changes in direction, speed merges into the concept of agility, which again is vital in many sports. The ability to move from position A to position B quickly allows the athlete to attain the correct position for the specific sports skill.[9] The inclusion of these factors in the rehabilitation programme will ensure that the athlete's performance, on returning to training and competition, is maintained or even improved.

Strength

Strengthening should be performed through range, be progressive in nature, and be specific to the requirements of the sport. A muscle should be strengthened concentrically and eccentrically.

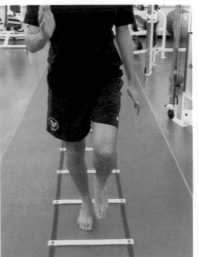

Agility activity using ladders in forwards position

The occurrence of injuries could be reduced if differences in muscle strengths were identified correctly and corrected. Many sports physiotherapists have realised the value of working very closely with strength and conditioning experts—not only in trying to improve the strength of an injured muscle but in generally maintaining global strength.

Methods for achieving strength
- Isokinetic machines
- Resistance bands
- Body weight
- Weight training with machines and free weights

Power
Power, also called speed strength, is crucial to many sports performers and should be developed as a separate component to strength, especially where acceleration is relevant to the sport specific skill. Conditioning programmes designed by the physiotherapist should be relevant, specific to the individual sport, and include all aspects of fitness and conditioning.[9]

Endurance
When an athlete is taken through the rehabilitation programme, one of the aims should be to maintain a certain amount of cardiovascular fitness. If the athlete is unable to run because of the injury, cycling or an aquajogger in the hydrotherapy pool can be used as an alternative. Improvement of the endurance of whole body movements as well as single joint movements is the responsibility of the attending physiotherapist, along with other sports science team members.

The ability to perform certain tasks—be they exercises or sports techniques—needs to be improved gradually in number and intensity. Endurance exercises need to be sport specific, as excessive exercises may well affect power negatively, which is important in certain sports

Skill
Skill not only includes the ability to perform the sporting action but also refers to regaining balance and coordination. In this respect, skill is a vital part of all stages of rehabilitation—ranging from walking with a reciprocal gait on crutches to being able to jump and land on one foot while performing an intricate sporting action. Sports physiotherapists should ensure that upper and lower limb injury rehabilitation programmes include proprioception and balance activities in the functional rehabilitation, with equipment such as wobbleboards and mini trampolines

Fitness testing

Before any injured athlete is allowed to return to training, they must have undergone some form of fitness test. An athlete should never be asked to "go and see how you get on" in training. Fitness testing is an ongoing procedure during the treatment and rehabilitation programme. No treatment progression is made without the physiotherapist having formally or informally appraised the level of improvement. As the athlete more closely attains the parameters of fitness mentioned previously, the rehabilitation progresses from the clinic to the gymnasium and eventually to the athlete's training environment (pitch, pool, court and so on). Fitness tests can be done in the clinic but are carried out more effectively at the training venue.

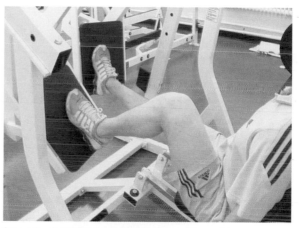
Strength rehabilitation—weight training with machines

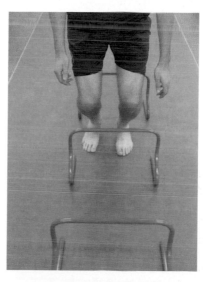
Improving power—using hurdles to introduce a plyometric aspect to rehabilitation

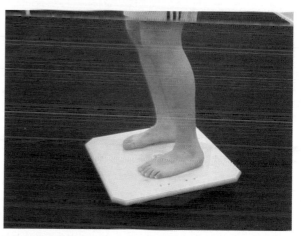
Rehabilitation programmes should include using equipment such as wobbleboards

Formal fitness test
All parameters must be tested fully, as a weakness in any aspect increases the risk of reinjury.

Athletes need to be tested under conditions that most closely replicate:
- Their position or event
- The physical and mental stress
- The length of time they are involved in activity (including repetitive events) during training and competition

Injury prevention

The physiotherapist's role is to prevent injury and reinjury as much as to treat injuries. Awareness is increasing of the value of identifying weaknesses and imbalances in the athlete's musculoskeletal system and correcting these in an attempt to prevent repetitive strain on certain areas resulting in an injury.

Profiling

Assessment of the musculoskeletal system by physiotherapists allows for identification and monitoring of the parameters of fitness mentioned above, including postural differences. In particular, changes that occur during growth spurts or intensive training can be monitored. Correction of identified problems could arguably lead to a reduction in injuries, but only if accompanied by a specific exercise programme that addresses the issues. Care is needed when changing an aspect of the athlete's musculoskeletal system that deviates from the expected "norm" because individual differences may represent an advantageous variant. Profiling is most valid if the assessing physiotherapist remains unchanged to maintain reliability.

Strapping and supports

Strapping is used commonly to prevent and protect injuries, especially in the ankle.[10] Strapping is thought to support the weakened area by providing an "external ligament" that increases the mechanical stability, reduces range of movement, and improves proprioceptive function.[11] Prophylactic taping of the ankle has been shown to be no more effective than coordination training of the ankle in the prevention of injuries.[12]

An accurate assessment of joints and soft tissues is needed before strapping is applied. Strapping should only be used as a substitute for normal soft tissue function and stability.[13] Strapping must never be seen as a substitute for treatment and rehabilitation.[14]

Neoprene braces are suggested to help maintain an increased skin temperature and thus an increased peripheral blood flow, which could be argued to help prevent injury. Some ankle braces have been shown adversely to affect ankle joint kinematics during landing.[15] This may or may not be something to consider when prescribing a supportive stabilising brace.

Education

Great value is gained by educating athlete and coach about warm up before competition and cool down after competition. Cooperation between all parties will increase awareness of potential injury risks that could lead to injury, such as overuse or repetitive forms of training. Athlete and coach need to be aware of the treatment being given by the medical team, as well as the time scales in which recovery may be achieved. Both parties again need to be made aware of the restrictions to training that are in place and when these may change. The dangers of not adhering to set time scales and parameters need to be clearly explained and discussed, as returning to activity too early can lead to reinjury and an extended recovery phase.

Performance enhancement

The ultimate goal of any physiotherapist is to return the injured athlete to competition, but the added goal of increasing performance should not be forgotten. By correctly rehabilitating an athlete (and after the performance restoration principle), the possibility exists of returning the athlete in a stronger state, enabling them to perform more effectively.

"Drawing a map" of the athlete's body helps track differences between left and right and identifies weaknesses between agonist and antagonist

Strapping and supports often are used in an attempt to get an athlete back into training more quickly. Arguably this is a risky philosophy, as research that suggests the role of strapping in preventing reinjury is limited

Although research into the value of strapping and braces is limited, sufficient anecdotal evidence warrants considering it as a treatment adjunct after an injury and during rehabilitation. As prophylaxis, they are less useful

1 Kerr KM, Daley LD, Booth L, Stark J. *Guidelines for the management of soft-tissue (musculoskeletal) injury with protection, rest, ice, compression and elevation (PRICE) during the first 72 hours*. London: Chartered Society of Physiotherapy, 1999
2 Maitland G. *Vertebral manipulation*. Oxford: Butterworth/Heinemann, 1996
3 Shrier I, Gossal K. Myths and truths of stretching. Individualised recommendations for healthy muscles. *Phys Sport Med* 2000;28:57-63
4 Anderson JC, Burke ER. Scientific, medical and practical aspects of stretching. *Clin Sport Med* 1991;10:63-86
5 Fees M, Decker T, Snyder-Mackler L, Axe MJ. Upper extremity weight-training modifications for the injured athlete. A clinical perspective. *Am J Sports Med* 1998;26:732-42
6 Knott M, Voss DE. *Proprioceptive neuromuscular facilitation: patterns and techniques*, 2nd edn. Philadelphia, PA: Harper and Row, 1968
7 Elphinston J, Pook P. *The core workout*. Cardiff: Core Workout, 1998
8 Bergmark A. Stability of the lumbar spine. A study in mechanical engineering. *Acta Orth Scand* 1996;230:20-4
9 Kraemer WJ, Fry AC. Strength testing: development and evaluation of methodology. In: *Physiological assessment of human fitness*. Moud P, Foster C (eds)
10 Fumich RM, Ellison AE, Guerin GJ, Grace PD. The measured effect of taping on combined foot and ankle motion before and after exercise. *Am J Sports Med* 1981;9:165-70
11 Karlsson J, Andreasson GO. The effect of external ankle support in chronic ankle joint instability. An electromyographic study. *Am J Sport Med* 1992;20:257-61
12 Tropp H, Askling C, Gillquist J. Prevention of ankle sprains. *Am J Sports Med* 1985;139:259-62
13 Karlsson J, Sward L, Andreasson GO. The effect of taping on ankle stability. *Sports Med* 1993;16:210-15
14 Macdonald R, ed. *Taping technique. Principles and practice*. Oxford: Butterworth/Heinemann, 1994
15 McCaw ST, Cerullo JF. Prophylactic ankle stabilizers affect ankle joint kinematics during drop landings. *Med Sci Sports Exercise* 1999;31:702-7

Further reading

● Perrin DH, ed. *The injured athlete*. New York and Philadelphia: Lippincott-Raven, 1999

22   Providing a "one stop shop" for sports medicine

Richard Godfrey

Improved funding for sport is causing a growth in the sports science and medicine services available to support high level and elite sport. The expertise, skills, and facilities to provide quality services that address the very specific needs of the high level performer are neither common nor extensive. Indeed even if they were, the task of funding individual experts who provide services from different venues around the country would be insurmountable.

Accordingly, the best way to provide services may be by establishing "oases" of elite service provision where athletes can access expert medical and scientific support at, or near training venues. This concept has led to institutes dedicated to specialist delivery of sports medicine and science being set up in key locations. What services should be on offer, and therefore what facilities are required are key questions in the provision of quality services.

Rationale for a "one stop shop"

The advantages of operating institutes that offer a range of disciplines are many and varied. The best quality of service occurs when time is managed appropriately and carefully, and selected staff members are experienced and confident in their own knowledge and ability so that they can defer to better qualified colleagues as necessary. However, there should be sufficient staff and enough contact time between them to encourage cross fertilisation of ideas, consultation, and interdisciplinary practice. Coordination of service delivery improves the efficacy of support by drawing on all facets of the support services in a multidisciplinary and interdisciplinary environment at the same time. The availability of training facilities at the institute may be valuable in the delivery of sport specific support. The one stop shop facilitates the best possible treatment and rehabilitation for the injured athlete where the possibility of a case conference approach can be used where appropriate. This could mean a physician, physiotherapist, psychologist, nutritionist, and physiologist would discuss a particular case with the athlete concerned, hence helping to minimise delay in diagnosis and treatment, and optimising the athlete's return to competitive fitness.

In addition, where an athlete is attending the institute for fitness assessment and advice, any minor medical or injury problem can be checked at the same time. Regular physiological profiling can provide a wealth of information on the baseline condition of the healthy athlete that is invaluable to the physician, physiotherapist, and psychologist when the athlete attends ill or injured on a subsequent occasion. Regular physiological profiling also allows identification of improvements in and weaknesses of physiology that can inform the coach and allow "fine tuning" of the training programme. Much debate remains around the issue of musculoskeletal and medical screening. It is clear, however, that specific, targeted screening programmes can be advantageous to injury or illness identification, tracking, and prevention.

Advantages of a "one stop shop"

- Availability of experts from a number of disciplines provides a greater guarantee of optimal strategies for improving rehabilitation, recovery, health, fitness, acclimatisation, and performance
- An athlete can have a number of issues relating to health and performance decrement at one time

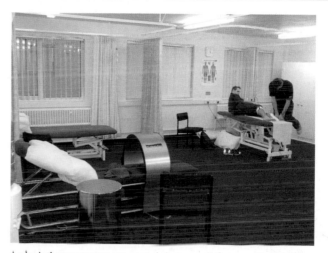

A physiotherapy treatment room is just one of the many facilities that should be available at a "one stop shop"

Case study 1: spontaneous atrial fibrillation in a freestyle skier

A 19 year old male freestyle skier presented for routine physiological assessment consisting of an incremental treadmill test to volitional exhaustion to ascertain VO_{2max}. After the test, the athlete's heart rate failed to fall as expected. Furthermore, the athlete complained of chest pain and shortness of breath. The athlete was then attached to a 12 lead electrocardiograph machine that showed atrial fibrillation with a ventricular rate of 155 beats per minute. An institute physician and the on call cardiologist were informed. The athlete was monitored for two hours, during which time the atrial fibrillation persisted and the athlete became compromised. Subsequently, the athlete was admitted to the coronary care unit, the atrial fibrillation was cardioverted successfully with flecainide (150 mg over 30 minutes), and after 24 hours of observation, the athlete was discharged.

On follow up examination, the athlete was in sinus rhythm and had a normal venous pulse and normal heart sounds. Echocardiography showed normal intracardiac dimensions with normal systolic function of left and right ventricles, and 24 hour electrocardiography showed sinus rhythm throughout. During integrated cardiopulmonary exercise stress testing, the athlete achieved a VO_{2max} of 53.5 ml/kg/min and a maximum heart rate of 201 beats per minute. No inducible arrhythmias were seen during or after exercise. During consultation, the athlete admitted consuming 12 units of alcohol (an excessive amount compared with his normal consumption) two days before the initial physiological assessment. The observed atrial fibrillation was diagnosed as a lone episode of alcohol induced atrial fibrillation, and the athlete was counselled about alcohol consumption and vigorous exercise.

Case study 2: diagnosis of McArdle's disease in a young hockey player

A 17 year old male naval recruit was referred by his medical officer to check whether his malaise, pain, and inability to keep up during long marches was part of an undiagnosed clinical condition.

The medical centre's clinician consultant requested routine physiological assessment. This consisted of an incremental treadmill test to volitional exhaustion to ascertain heart rate profile, lactate profile and VO_{2max}. Five submaximal incremental stages were completed before the patient had to stop because of pain. The highest VO_2 achieved was around 40 ml/kg/min and the respiratory exchange ratio was around 0.7—unusual this far into an incremental test. On cessation, a heart rate of 198 beats per minute was recorded, consistent with age predicted maximum, and lactate values started at 1.2 mmol/l, fluctuated only a little ($+0.3$ mmol/l) between increments, and was 0.4 mmol/l at the end of exercise. Discussion led the physiologist and doctor to a speculative conclusion of metabolic dysfunction. A biopsy sample taken from the vastus lateralis and stained with periodic acid Schiff for muscle carbohydrate, showed an abnormally large preponderance of muscle glycogen.

Analysis of DNA showed the subject to be "r49x/r49x," that is, homozygous for a missense mutation to arginine at codon 49 in intron 1; hence the gene for myophosphorylase had been deleted. Myophosphorylase initiates the degradation of muscle glycogen that normally leads to the production of pyruvate, lactate and the formation of the useable form of energy, ATP. Hence in the absence of this key enzyme glycolysis doesn't occur, lactate is not formed and energy production from this substrate cannot occur. This impairs exercise capacity, results in muscle pain and contracture and can lead to myoglobinuria with renal failure as a possible outcome. This is McArdle's disease, type V glycogen storage disease. The patient was discharged from the Navy and was restricted to low level exercise from then on. This shows the role exercise physiology can play in helping the clinician find the most appropriate follow up and in making an accurate diagnosis.

What facilities should be available?

A good sports science and medicine institute should have the following facilities:

- Fully equipped medical consulting room
- Physiotherapy treatment room
- Rehabilitation gym
- Aquatherapy room
- Nutrition consulting room
- Psychology consulting room
- Air conditioned physiology laboratory
- Seminar room
- Accommodation
- Good links with NHS or private hospitals to facilitate "fast tracking" for diagnostics and more serious medical problems, particularly orthopaedic facilities.

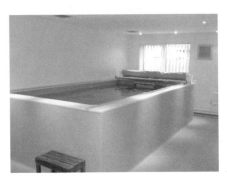

Aquatherapy pool

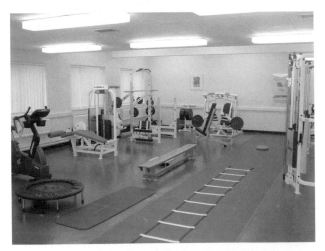

Rehabilitation gymnasium

Which services should be available?

The following services should be available:

- Medicine—general, respiratory, haematology, cardiology, orthopaedic, rheumatology, gynaecology, dermatology, fast tracking of acute problems, and tertiary referral
- Physiotherapy—soft tissue injury treatment, orthopaedic treatment, acupuncture, hydrotherapy, and tertiary referral
- Biomechanics—gait analysis and notational analysis and advice
- Nutrition—dietary analysis and advice and shopping and cooking advice and instruction

---

Case study 3: interdisciplinary team in rehabilitation of a tibial fracture

A 22 year old female marathon runner was diagnosed with a tibial fracture and began an in house rehabilitation programme in a residential sports science institute. Consultation with a psychologist was used throughout to minimise the likelihood of negative mental imagery and development of mental programmes that might hinder the rehabilitation process.

A sports dietitian conducted a dietary analysis and prepared a menu planner to ensure optimal nutrition for the duration. The dietitian also spent time with the athlete, providing tuition in buying and cooking appropriate food for optimal sports nutrition. The physiotherapist and strength and conditioning specialist drew up an exercise programme that began with a substantial volume of deep water running in the aquatherapy pool and upper body resistance exercise in the gymnasium.

Throughout the rehabilitation period, increasing amounts of land work were added to the programme. This began with some cycling exercise and increased until exercise loaded to normal body weight was possible.

In six weeks, the athlete was ready to be retested in the laboratory (initial testing had occurred, coincidentally, a few weeks before the injury). Before the injury, VO_{2max} was 66 ml/kg/min and lactate threshold occurred at a VO_2 equivalent to 67% of VO_{2max}. After rehabilitation, VO_{2max} was 71 ml/kg/min and lactate threshold as a percentage of VO_{2max} was 74%. Body mass and fat levels had remained relatively unchanged.

This shows that appropriate action taken by an interdisciplinary team in a one stop shop setting should be able to at least maintain the fitness of the athlete during the rehabilitation period or even slightly improve their fitness.

- Psychology—skills associated with occupational, clinical, and sports psychology are recommended; these can provide skill acquisition advice and learning of mental skills (such as attention and anxiety control)
- Physiology—laboratory based service should include sport specific ergospirometry, lactate profiling, cardiopulmonary assessment, and strength and power testing; field based service should include monitoring during domestic training sessions and domestic and overseas training camps.

A few considerations

Medicine and physiotherapy

The most important aspect is a general practice service in which each doctor providing the role has specialist sports medicine training. This accommodates the two most common and important areas of acute illness and injury. A fast track service that can provide appropriate rapid care for serious problems is rare in the United Kingdom and is one area in which improvements in the provision of care could make a huge impact. The Olympic Medical Institute is based at Northwick Park Hospital, and so has access to all of the services (including imaging and surgery) that are common at a large general hospital.

In most cases the most important issue is reducing the athlete's down time as a result of illness or injury, hence minimising the magnitude of deconditioning. Medical and physiotherapy services should be conducted with this in mind. The presence of physiologists, strength and conditioning specialists, nutritionist, and psychologists can increase the speed of the recovery process.

Physiology

Laboratory based testing provides a standardised means of collecting information on and reviewing the current state of health and conditioning of the athlete, so it is verifiable and objective. Despite the use of sports specific ergometry, it is rare to reproduce an ecologically valid test in the laboratory. Field based testing allows physiological assessment to occur in the environment in which training and competition occurs—using the same equipment in exactly the same way it would be used in training and competition. Field based testing is more sports specific and thus has greater ecological validity, but it is also more subjective, as it is difficult to standardise data collection. The best solution is one that recognises the relative strengths and weaknesses of field and laboratory based testing and so uses both to advantage. One acts as an adjunct to, and often eliminates the deficiencies of, the other. In practice, a knowledge of the sport helps determine the number of times laboratory and field based testing should occur. For an endurance sport (like marathon running), three or four laboratory tests may be needed per year, whereas only one may be needed for high intensity or explosive sports (like polevaulting).

Field based support

Decisions on what physiological support occurs at training camps depends largely on where the camp is (*viz* altitude, weather conditions, global location, whether jet lag is a major issue) and when the camp takes place (the camp could be a routine training camp or a precompetition preparation camp). Support is the testing or monitoring in a field based setting. Testing generally involves collecting data during the athlete's sporting activity, and the aim is to identify or verify training zones. Monitoring athletes in the field usually refers to daily, early morning monitoring. It is designed to examine the athlete's health within the context of imposition of a further stress caused by living in a challenging environment

An interdisciplinary system drawing upon physiology and medicine resulted in rapid identification and treatment and as a result a fast return to competition. In addition, the experience informed the physiological assessment of athletes, indicating a role for electrocardiogram monitoring during routine testing

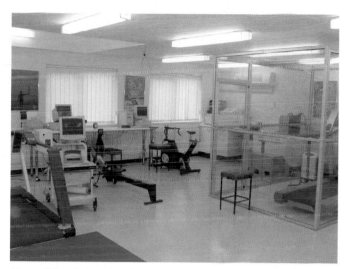

Air conditioned physiology laboratory

Summary of typical laboratory based assessment

- Height, weight, and skin fold measurement for body composition profiling
- Isokinetic strength testing, rebound jumping, and Wingate test for power profiling, with appropriate sports specific tests selected
- Incremental test to maximum for lactate profiling and assessment of maximal oxygen consumption with appropriate sports specific equipment and protocols
- Flow volume loop testing to assess respiratory function

Summary of typical field based support

Testing
- Incremental sports specific test to establish heart rate associated with lactate threshold or confirmation of suitability of laboratory derived heart rate zones for field based sports specific training
- Measurement of lactate serially immediately after competition to ensure warm down efficacy

Monitoring
- Early morning heart rate, body weight, urine concentration, and blood urea concentration to monitor relative stress of training and avoid subsequent unexplained underperformance syndrome
- Early morning administration of a psychology or multidisciplinary inventory

Medical priorities for a sports medicine institute

- General practitioners with qualifications and experience in specialist sports medicine
- Fast track system, preferably on site at the institute

Accreditation, calibration, quality control, and quality assessment

Accreditation

National and international professional associations produce guidelines for standards of facilities and practice. The British Association of Sport and Exercise Sciences (BASES) has an accreditation system which checks and "certifies" the competencies of individual physiologists and checks and "certifies" the standard of exercise physiology laboratories and the methods employed within them.

Calibration

Following standardised calibration procedures regularly is important. For example, the force transducer for a rowing ergometer may be calibrated with a range of known masses before and after every 20 rowers tested. Oxygen and carbon dioxide analysers should be calibrated before and after testing each athlete. This is performed by testing a certified gas of known concentration in the analysers. A lactate analyser may be calibrated after every 10 samples by testing a solution containing a standardised concentration of lactate and, if necessary, altering the lactate analyser's acceptance of a given concentration relative to the standard. Records of calibrations, and particularly any problems with calibration and their solution, should be kept.

Validity and reliability

A recognised, validated means of assessing validity and reliability of a given parameter should be used and records should be kept. The reproducibility of measuring oxygen consumption with an online gas analysis system should, for example, be measured, as should its comparison against the accepted "gold standard" Douglas bag measurement, and the difference between them should be no more than 2% (British Association of Sport and Exercise Sciences guidelines, 1993). If a different means of assessment is to be used, for example measuring lactate in the field not the laboratory, comparisons should be made and information used accordingly. For example, if the field device for lactate measurement routinely overpredicts or underpredicts when compared with a laboratory based analyser, a correction factor can be calculated. If variable overprediction or underprediction occurs, data from the field and laboratory cannot be used interchangeably. In this case, it is best to adopt a different field based device that allows correction against the laboratory based system.

Physiological priorities for a medicine and science institute

- Provision of both laboratory and field based services
- Laboratory and individual staff should be accredited to National or International professional body Standards (for example, BASES)
- All physiology staff should have a recent cardiopulmonary resuscitation certificate (for example, from the Resuscitation Council)
- Sports specific ergometers should be used in the laboratory
- The means to determine profiles of lactate and heart rate and maximal oxygen consumption
- The means to determine strength and power
- The means to assess body composition
- The means to provide written feedback from laboratory or field based testing within five working days

---

Further reading

- British Association of Sport and Exercise Sciences. *Guidelines to exercise testing.* Leeds: British Association of Sport and Exercise Sciences, 1993
- Australian Institute of Sport. *Guidelines to exercise testing.* Canberra: Australian Institute of Sport, 2002
- American College of Sports Medicine. *ACSM's guidelines to exercise testing.* Boston: American College of Sports Medicine, 2000

23 Drugs in sport

Roger Palfreeman

In 1998, after a period of undercover surveillance, French customs officers stopped and searched a team car during the Tour de France cycle race. Inside, they found a large number of doping products, including erythropoietin and growth hormone, which presumably were destined for use by the team's riders. A number of team officials and riders were subsequently questioned by the police, and the team's doctor, among others, ultimately was imprisoned for trafficking doping agents.

Other raids during professional cycling races were carried out that year and a coordinated response to the problem of doping clearly was required. In 1999, the World Anti-Doping Agency was established. In 2004, the World Anti-Doping Agency published its current list of prohibited substances, and this has now been adopted by most sports, although each sport may make slight modifications to the list according to its own needs. If any athlete has a medical need for any of the listed products, they must first obtain a therapeutic use exemption certificate. This applies for many commonly used drugs, such as asthma inhalers and steroid creams, for which an abbreviated application process for an abbreviated therapeutic use exemption certificate is available.

Substances prohibited in competition

Stimulants

For most stimulants, the mere presence of the compound in a urine sample denotes a positive test. In the case of ephedrine, the threshold limit is 10 μg/ml; methylephedrine has a threshold limit of 5 μg/ml.

In contrast with past years, caffeine, pseudoephedrine, and several other mild stimulants have been taken off the proscribed list and placed onto a monitoring programme, in which the World Anti-Doping Agency will continue to test for these substances to detect any pattern of misuse. If evidence of abuse emerges, such as very high urinary concentrations, the World Anti-Doping Agency reserves the right to return them to the proscribed list. Although this approach has been criticised, particularly in the case of caffeine, it reflects the fact that most positive tests for stimulants have come from inadvertent administration in over the counter drugs taken to relieve minor ailments.

Narcotics

Narcotics are proscribed because of their potential for dependence and harm to the athlete rather than any ergogenic effect. They can also be used to mask the pain of injuries with the attendant risk of further damage.

Cannabinoids

Cannabinoids (for example, cannabis) are prohibited, once again, because of their potential to cause harm rather than any sporting advantage.

Anabolic agents

Anabolic androgenic steroidal agents
This category includes a large number of steroid compounds, the most notable currently being nandrolone (19-nortestosterone) and tetrahydrogestrinone (THG). Low levels of nandrolone are produced naturally in the body, and, for this reason, threshold values of 2 ng/ml and 5 ng/ml have been set for men and women, respectively. Over the past few years, a

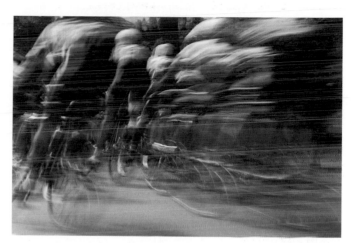

In 1998 raids took place during professional cycle races, and it quickly became apparent that drug abuse in sport was taking place on a scale previously not imagined

World Anti-Doping Agency

The World Anti-Doping Agency's remit was to coordinate a worldwide response to doping by working with governments, public authorities, and other involved bodies, such as:

- International sports federations
- National anti-doping organisations
- International Olympic Committee

The complete list of drugs prohibited by the World Anti-Doping Agency can be downloaded from their website (www.wada-ama.org/en/t1.asp). Professionals working in competitive sport should have a copy of this document

Stimulants

- Amphetamine
- Methylamphetamine
- Substances often found in over the counter cold remedies, such as:
  Ephedrine
  Methylephedrine

Narcotics

Proscribed narcotics include potent opioids, such as:
- Morphine
- Pethidine
- Diamorphine

Permitted narcotics include:
- Dihydrocodeine
- Codeine
- Pholcodine
- Other weak opioids

Anabolic steroids

- Precursors of nandrolone and testosterone often are found in nutritional supplements
- Levels of these contaminants are capable of producing a positive dope test
- Use of nutritional supplements should be monitored carefully and avoided wherever possible

large number of tests have been positive for levels of metabolites of nandrolone above the allowed level. Many athletes proclaim their innocence and attribute the findings to contaminated nutritional supplements. As a result, the International Olympic Committee recently studied a large number of nutritional supplements from 13 different countries—all supposedly free of any steroid compounds according to their product labelling. Of the 634 samples analysed, 94 (14.8%) contained prohormones of testosterone or nandrolone. The positive supplements contained steroid concentrations ranging from 0.01 µg to 190 µg/g of product. Excretion studies showed that a total intake of only 1 µg of prohormones of nandrolone produced urinary metabolite concentrations that exceeded the allowed levels for several hours. When the most highly contaminated supplement was taken in the recommended dose, the highest urinary concentration achieved was 623 ng/ml.

The products responsible for these results have not been named but included protein powders, creatine, carnitine, zinc, vitamins, minerals, and herbal extracts. It seems likely that at least some tests positive for nandrolone are because of inadvertent administration of prohormones (19-norandrostenedione and 19-norandrostenediol) contained in commonly used supplements. More potent steroids, such as methanedienone (Dianabol) also have been discovered, which raises the possibility that some manufacturers may be deliberately manipulating their products to cause greater effects in users, thus increasing sales.

Non-steroidal anabolic agents

Just two drugs fall into this subcategory—clenbuterol and zeranol—and both have been used as growth promoters in the beef industry. Clenbuterol is a β_2 agonist that also is used in the treatment of asthma in people in some countries of the European Community but not in the United Kingdom. Clenbuterol first came to prominence just before the 1992 Olympics Games in Barcelona, when two British weightlifters tested positive. Zeranol is a non-steroidal oestrogen analogue that is only for veterinary use.

Peptide hormones

Peptide hormones account for many of the products known to be widely abused in a variety of different sports. It also includes their mimetics, analogues and releasing factors.

Recombinant human erythropoietin—erythropoietin is a glycoprotein hormone produced by the kidney. It acts on erythroid precursors in the bone marrow to increase the rate of red blood cell production, thus improving the ability of the blood to transport oxygen. In the late 1980s, recombinant (synthetic) erythropoietin became available, and its use by professional road cyclists and cross country skiers, in particular, became widespread. By the mid to late 1990s, evidence showed that some professional cyclists were riding with a haematocrit of up to 65%—similar to that of residents at extreme high altitudes. Furthermore, this use of erythropoietin often was accompanied by intravenous iron infusions, in the belief that oral iron supplementation was not enough to support such accelerated rates of erythrocyte formation. Iron overload became common, with ferritin levels often in excess of 1000 ng/ml—similar to the levels seen in patients who have hereditary haemochromatosis. Detection of recombinant human erythropoietin use currently involves the use of two complementary methods. Given the current difficulties faced by the antidoping authorities, the sports of cross country skiing and cycling have taken a pragmatic approach and set upper threshold limits for haematocrit before competition.

Tetrahydrogestrinone

Tetrahydrogestrinone is a new steroid compound that has been discovered recently. It is similar structurally to gestrinone, which is used to treat endometriosis.

In 2003, the existence of this new steroid was brought to the attention of the United States' Anti-Doping Agency, which subsequently arranged for retesting of a number of urine samples recently obtained from prominent athletes. Evidence of the use of tetrahydrogestrinone was found in several cases.

Tetrahydrogestrinone has been alleged to represent just one of a range of "designer drugs" that have been engineered chemically to try to evade detection by drug testing.

> Some evidence from animal studies shows that clenbuterol can produce anabolic effects on muscle and reduce adipose tissue through its action at β_2 receptors. The doses used in these studies, however, were far higher than those that people are able to tolerate, and the effects on humans are less certain

Peptide hormones

- Erythropoietin
- Growth hormone and insulin like growth factor
- Chorionic gonadotrophin (prohibited in men only)
- Pituitary and synthetic gonadotrophins (prohibited in men only)
- Insulin
- Corticotrophins

Recombinant human erythropoietin

- Widely abused in endurance sports
- Still difficult to detect its use, despite tests being available
- Setting upper limits for haematocrit is a crude but effective way of limiting erythropoietin's use
- New types of recombinant human erythropoietin that are even more difficult to detect are now available

Detection of recombinant human erythropoietin

Indirect method

This method requires a small blood sample and examines various haematological indices of red cell production, including reticulocyte count and levels of erythropoietin in serum. Current (ON model) and recent (OFF model) use of rhEPO can be shown with a very high degree of accuracy

Direct method

As false positives can occasionally occur with the indirect method, a second, more complicated and more specific test that relies on the detection of recombinant human erythropoietin fragments in a urine sample is used. Unfortunately, this test, pioneered in the French National Anti-Doping Laboratory, has relatively low sensitivity. Out of 20 "anomalous" urine samples taken from riders in the 2003 Tour de France, only one finally could be declared unequivocally positive, even though the other 19 showed evidence of using recombinant human erythropoietin

If a competitor's haematocrit exceeds these values (50% and 47% for men and women, respectively), they are withdrawn from competing for at least 14 days and until their readings fall below the upper normal limit. Competitors with naturally high haematocrits may undergo further testing and obtain special dispensation to return higher readings.

Growth hormone and insulin like growth factor—these two related products are thought to be abused widely by strength and endurance athletes. The general belief is that they are effective in building muscle and reducing adipose tissue. Very little evidence, however, supports an anabolic action for either drug used in isolation. In practice, they are used often along with insulin or anabolic steroids, so their true effect remains unknown. Beyond doubt is their potential for adverse effects, including permanent skeletal changes and cardiomyopathy. Furthermore, as most human recombinant growth hormone is obtained on the black market, the product supplied is not guaranteed to contain any active hormone. In some cases, inactive bovine growth hormone or human chorionic gonadotrophin are substituted. More worrying is the discovery that some growth hormones packaged as recombinant (synthetic) growth hormone actually contain hormone obtained from the pituitary glands of cadavers, which raises the prospect of transmission of Creutzfeldt Jakob disease to the unwitting user. No validated method of detection exists for either substance.

Insulin—may be ergogenic through its inhibition of protein degradation and probably acts synergistically with growth hormone to generate an anabolic effect. In addition, it promotes muscle glycogen synthesis secondary to increased glucose uptake, which may help explain why it is used by endurance athletes, such as professional road cyclists when they are competing in stage races. Insulin is only allowed in diabetics, who must first obtain a therapeutic use exemption.

Corticotrophins—tetracosactide (Synacthen) consists of the first 24 N-terminal amino acids of adrenocorticotropic hormone. It is given by injection and acts on the adrenal cortex to promote secretion of glucocorticosteroids. The plasma half life of tetracosactide is in the order of a few minutes, which makes detection extremely difficult. It is used primarily in endurance sports instead of or as an adjunct to systemic corticosteroids.

β_2 agonists—salbutamol, salmeterol, and terbutaline are allowed only by inhalation to prevent asthma and exercise induced bronchoconstriction. Even when a therapeutic use exemption has been granted for use of an asthma inhaler, urinary concentrations of salbutamol > 1000 ng/ml are considered positive (as an anabolic agent), as such levels are extremely unlikely to result from anything but systemic use.

Agents with anti-oestrogenic activity—these are prohibited only in men, where they are used to counter the oestrogenic side effects of anabolic steroids, principally gynaecomastia.

Masking agents—some chemically unrelated substances are used to hide the presence of banned substances. Examples include plasma expanders, such as hydroxyethyl starch, or human albumin solution, which can lower the haematocrit transiently in people who have been using recombinant human erythropoietin. This allows the user to fall below the haematocrit limits set in certain sports.

Glucocorticosteroids—permitted for use topically, such as through asthma inhalers and skin creams, as well as by intra-articular or soft tissue injection. Systemic corticosteroids are banned and probably are abused widely in some endurance sports, where they are used for a number of reasons.

Darbepoietin and epoietin delta

A long acting form of human recombinant erythropoietin, called darbepoietin, has become available recently. This allows patients with renal problems (and unscrupulous athletes) to reduce the frequency of administration. The long half life and molecular modification, however, makes its detection as a doping agent relatively easy.

Unfortunately, the same cannot be said for epoietin delta (marketed as Dynepo). Unlike the original recombinant human erythropoietins, this is produced entirely in human cell lines, which likely renders it undetectable by the "gold standard" urinary test for erythropoietin. Until the blood tests for human recombinant erythropoietin are refined further and are accepted as definitive proof of abuse of this drug, this situation is unlikely to change.

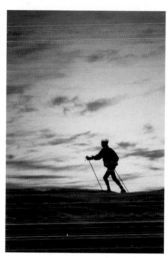

The sport of cross country skiing has set upper threshold limits for haematocrit before competition

Growth hormone

- Used by strength and endurance athletes
- Little evidence of anabolic action exists
- Potential for severe side effects
- Detection methods are still under research

Reasons for use of glucocorticosteroids

- Anecdotally, they are thought to result in the breakdown of adipose tissue, particularly when combined with high volumes of endurance training
- They also promote the use of lipids as fuel during exercise, resulting in sparing of muscle and liver glycogen
- High doses may potentiate the effects of catecholamines on the cardiovascular system, thereby producing a secondary sympathomimetic effect

Limited research evidence supports these suggestions; however, their widespread use in some endurance activities cannot be challenged—60% of cyclists who were tested for doping in the 2003 Tour de France declared the use of non-systemic corticosteroids in their health records. A large discrepancy was noted, however, between the high levels of drug found in urine samples and the timing and route of administration recorded by the rider. Suspicion was strong that prescriptions for common corticosteroid preparations were being used as a cover for systemic injection. Further research into this area has been proposed by the World Anti-Doping Agency.

Tetracosactide, although not actually a corticosteroid itself, promotes the release of endogenous substances such as cortisol and likely has similar effects

Methods prohibited in competition

Enhancement of oxygen transfer

Blood doping
Blood doping is the infusion of cross matched blood from a donor (homologous) or reinfusion of stored red cells previously taken from the circulation (autologous) after a delay of several weeks to allow the bone marrow to replenish the "donated" red blood cells. These techniques largely became redundant after the development of recombinant human erythropoietin, but with the advent of tests capable of detecting use of recombinant human erythropoietin, these practices have re-emerged.

Use of products that enhance oxygen transfer
Haemoglobin based oxygen carriers—contain non-cellular haemoglobin of bovine, human, or recombinant origin. The most advanced product is Hemopure, which is licensed in South Africa for the treatment of acute blood loss. Early studies indicated it may be very effective as a doping agent—at least during submaximal exercise intensities—however, despite evidence of its abuse in sport, any potential ergogenic benefit may be lost at workloads approaching VO_{2max} because of its potent vasoconstrictor effect. Recent use of Hemopure can now be detected in a blood sample.

Perfluorocarbons—synthetic emulsions that readily dissolve oxygen. The most promising is currently in phase 3 trials. Their main limitation is the need to inspire high partial pressures of oxygen in order to dissolve large amounts in the perfluorocarbon molecule. Even so, the small increase in oxygen carrying capacity obtained when ambient air is breathed may still enhance performance. Perfluorocarbon can be detected in blood or expired air, although the test is only included in doping controls in exceptional circumstances.

Allosteric haemoglobin effectors—used to treat hyperlipidaemia. They act by stabilising the deoxygenated form of haemoglobin, which facilitates oxygen offloading. Efaproxiral (RSR13) shows most promise and is currently involved in a number of phase 3 clinical trials as a potential treatment for acute coronary syndromes and cerebrovascular events and as a radiosensitising agent in cancer therapy. Unlike haemoglobin based oxygen carriers, efaproxiral causes vasodilatation in the vascular bed of exercising muscles and thus has greater potential for use as a doping agent. The risk that it will be abused in endurance sports is obvious, and a detection method based on a urine sample already has been developed.

Pharmacological, chemical, and physical manipulation

This refers to the use of methods or substances that alter the integrity of the urine or blood samples. It includes urine substitution, reducing renal excretion of proscribed drugs, and altering testosterone or epitestosterone ratios.

Gene doping

The erythropoietin gene can already be introduced into cells that do not produce erythropoietin in other primates. When this was performed on baboons, however, the haematocrit rose rapidly from 40% to 75% in the space of 10 weeks, and regular venesection was then needed to prevent death. Similar experiments have been carried out with the growth hormone gene. The main limitation to the use of such technology in humans is the subsequent lack of control over hormone production. Once this barrier has been removed, we might see such methods used in sport. The hormones produced by genetically modified cells would effectively be endogenous in origin and extremely difficult to detect.

Detection of blood doping

Homologous transfusions involve erythrocytes that are cross-matched for ABO and Rhesus (D) compatibility but not usually for minor blood group antigens. Such "foreign" antigens now can be identified at least four weeks after administration, making this method of blood doping relatively easy to detect

Unfortunately, no definitive method for detecting autologous transfusions exists

Key points

- Most sports have now adopted the World Anti-Doping Agency code. All those working in competitive sport should make themselves familiar with it
- Many common over-the-counter medicines contain proscribed substances
- A number of nutritional supplements have been shown to be contaminated by precursors of testosterone and nandrolone
- Competitive sportspeople should keep their use of such supplements to an absolute minimum to avoid the possibility of an inadvertent positive dope test
- The detection of banned substances and methods is improving, but several areas of weakness still exist

Further reading

- Mottram DR, ed. *Drugs in sport*. New York: Routledge, 2003
- Gaudard A, Varlet-Marie E, Berssolle F, Audran M. Drugs for increasing oxygen transport and their potential use in doping. *Sports Med* 2003;33:187-212
- Rennie MJ. Claims for the anabolic effects of growth hormone: a case of the Emperor's new clothes? *Br J Sports Med* 2003;37:100-5
- Schumacher YO, Schmid A, Dinkelmann S, Berg A, Northoff H. Artificial Oxygen Carriers—the new doping threat in endurance sport? *Int J Sports Med* 2001;22:566-71
- Jenkins P. Growth hormone and exercise. *Clin Endocrinol* 1999;50:683-9
- Schanzer W. Analysis of non-hormonal nutritional supplements for androgenic anabolic steroids. International Olympic Committee report, 2002
- World Anti-Doping Agency. Independent Observer Report— Tour de France 2003
- Geyer H, Bredehoft M, Marek U, Parr MK, Schanzer W. High doses of the anabolic steroid Metandienone found in dietary supplements. *Eur J Sports Sciences* 2003;3:1-5
- Peltre G, Thorman W. Evaluation report of the EPO blood tests. World Anti-Doping Agency report, 2003
- Nelson M, Popp H, Sharpe K, Ashenden M. Proof of homologous blood transfusion through quantification of blood group antigens. *Haematologica* 2003;88:1284-95
- Leigh-Smith S. Blood boosting. *Br J Sports Med* 2004;38:99-101

Index

Notes: Page references in *italics* refer to figures, tables and boxed material.

Index

Index

Index

Index

middle third facial fractures 19, *19*
mid growth spurt 29
migraine with aura, diving 75
mineral supplements 84
mixed gas scuba diving 74
mobilisation, by physiotherapists 103
mobilised teeth 17
mobility, physiotherapy treatment 102
molluscum contagiosum 42, *42*
mometasone 38
mood monitoring, daily *48*
motor vehicle crashes *8*
mountain climbing
   disabled athletes 76
   traumatic brain injury 8
mountain sickness, acute *58, 65*
mouth guards
   concussion prevention 11
   dental injury prevention 17
multiple sclerosis 79
muscle fibre types 82, *82*
muscular dystrophy 79
muscular endurance *93*
muscular strength (power) *93*
musculoskeletal injuries
   risk in new exercisers *96*
   spinal cord lesion athletes 78
musculoskeletal screening 107
musculoskeletal system, physiotherapist assessment 106
musculotendinous injuries, groin pain 24, *24*, 27, *27*
myocarditis, viral 40, 47
myositis ossificans in children 31, *31*

nail infections 43
nandrolone 111, 112
narcotics 111, *111*
nasopharyngeal airway tube 5
National Food Survey, obesity 87
National Longitudinal Survey of Youth,
   childhood obesity 87, *87*
National Occupation Standards 100
natriuresis in divers 71
nebulised β_2 agonists 7
neck muscle conditioning 12
negative energy balance 81, *82*
neoprene braces, injury prevention 106
nerve entrapment, groin pain 25, *25*
neural tension 103
neurocardiogenic (vasovagal) syncope 56
neurological examination in concussion 10
neuropsychological tests in concussion 10, *10*, 11
nifedipine *65*, 78
nitric oxide 68
nitrogen, diving 72, *72*, 73
nitrogen dioxide 68
nitrogen narcosis 73, 74
nitrox, scuba diving 74
non-brain head injury 14–15
non-freezing injury 63–4, *64*
non-penetrating brain injury (closed head injury) 8
non-steroidal anabolic agents 112
non-steroidal anti-inflammatory drugs 7
nose
   fracture 17
   septal haematoma 16
nutrition *80*, 80–6
   sports science and medicine institute service 108
   strategies *83*, 83–4
      after exercise 84, *84*
      before exercise *83*, 83–4
      during exercise 84, *84*
   supplements *see* nutritional supplements

nutritional supplements 80, 84–5
   amino acids *84*, 84–5
   bicarbonate loading 85, *85*
   caffeine 85
   contamination with banned substances 112
   creatine 85, *85*
   minerals 84
   vitamins 84

obesity 87–8
   causes 87–8
   diabetes association 88, *88*
   prevalence 87, *87*
obturator hernia 24
obturator nerve entrapment 25
octopush 71
oestrogen replacement 53
olecranon apophysitis injury *33*
olecranon epiphysis fracture 33
olecranon physis stress reaction 34
oligomenorrhoea 50
Olympic Medical Institute 37, 109
Olympic Movement Anti-Doping Code 79
open fractures 15
Orchard sports injury classification system 2, *2*
orienteers, Swedish 40
oropharyngeal airway tube 5
Osgood-Schlatter's disease 32, *32*
osteitis pubis 25, 26, 27
osteoarthrosis, articular fractures in children 31
osteochondral fractures 31
osteochondritis dissecans in children 33, *33*
osteochondrosis in children 30
   articular 33, *33, 34*
   growth plate 34, *34*
   spinal 34, *34*
osteopenia 51–2
osteoporosis 50, 51–2
otitis externa 43
over drinking *84*
over-reaching 46, *46, 47*
overtraining syndrome *see* unexplained underperformance
   syndrome (overtraining syndrome)
overuse injuries
   in children *see* childhood injury management, overuse
      skeletal injuries
   disabled athletes participation risk *77*
   elderly 99
   groin disruption 25
   tendon injuries 24
oxidative stress 69, 70
oxides of nitrogen pollution 68, *68*
oxygen
   maximum consumption *see* $\dot{V}O_{2max}$
   partial pressures whilst diving 72, *72*
   scuba diving 73, *73*, 74
   toxicity, scuba diving 73
oxygen transfer enhancement 114
ozone pollution 68, *69*, 69–70, *70*

pacemakers, diving risk 75
pain reduction 102, *102*
Panner's disease 33
Paralympic games 77
paramedic crews 4, *4*
   see also immediate care
paraplegic athletes 76
   see also disability in sport
pars intra-articularis, stress fracture 34, *34*
participation risk
   disability in sport 76–7, *77*
   exercise for health benefit 95–6

Index

Index

vitamin E 70
vitamins, unexplained underperformance syndrome 48
vitamin supplements 84
vitreous haemorrhage 21
$\dot{V}O_{2max}$
   altitude effect 65
   cold water immersion effect 62
   energy metabolism 82
   exercise intensity monitoring 94–5
   in hot climates 59

walking, elderly 98
warm down 98, 106
warm up 98, 106
warts (verrucas) 42
water aerobics, elderly *97*
weight loss
   for competition 81
   exercise 88–9
wheelchair
   basketball 76, 78

dance 77
   marathon 76
   road racing 76
   sprint racing 76
wind chill *64*
wobbleboards 105, *105*
workplace exercise programme *89*
World Anti-Doping Agency 111, *111*
World Anti-Doping Code list (2004) 79
wounds, immediate care 7
wrestling
   hepatitis B 41
   herpes simplex virus 42
   weight loss for competition 81
wrist radiograph 29

yellow fever vaccine *45*
YMCA 100

zeranol 112
zygomatic (cheekbone) fractures 17–18, *18*

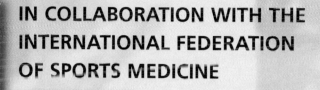
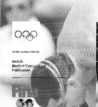
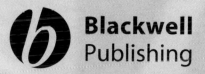